A GUIDE

FOR

EMERGENCIES

CONTAINING THE

HOMŒOPATHIC TREATMENT

OF SUCH DISEASES AS REQUIRE IMMEDIATE ATTENTION, AND OF SUCH AS MAY BE TREATED WITHOUT THE ASSISTANCE OF A PHYSICIAN; AND ALSO CONTAINING THE TREATMENT OF CASES OF POISONING, AND OF EVERY COMMON VARIETY OF ACCIDENTS.

FOR THE USE OF FAMILIES.

THIRD EDITION.

BY

HENRY B. MILLARD, M.D., A.M.,

LATE PROFESSOR OF THE PRACTICE OF MEDICINE IN THE NEW-YORK MEDICAL COLLEGE AND HOSPITAL FOR WOMEN, ETC.; AUTHOR OF "THE CLIMATE AND STATISTICS OF CONSUMPTION;" TRANSLATOR AND EDITOR OF "REIL ON ACONITE."

NEW-YORK:

PUBLISHED BY CHARLES T. HURLBURT,

No. 898 Broadway.

1871.

LIST OF REMEDIES PRESCRIBED.

REMEDIES.	ABBREVIATIONS.
Aconite	Ac.
Aloes	Al.
Arsenicum alb	Ars.
Belladonna	Bell.
Bryonia alb	Bry.
Chamomilla	Cham.
Colchicum	Colch.
Colocynth	Col.
Dulcamara	Dulc.
Euphrasia	Euph.
Gelseminum	Gel.
Hamamelis virg	Ham.
Hepar sulpharis	Hepar.
Hyoscyamus	Hyos.
Ignatia	Ig.
Ipecacuanha	Ipecac.
Jalapa	Jal.
Kali bichromate	Kali bich.
Kali hydriod	Kali h.
Mercurius corrosivus	Merc. c.
Mercurius dulcis	Merc. dul
Mercurius protiodide	Merc. prot.
Mercurius solubilis	Merc. sol.
Nux vomica	Nux.
Opium	Op.
Phosphorus	Phos.
Podophyllum	Pod.
Pulsatilla	Puls.
Rheum	Rheum.
Rhus. tox	Rhus.
Sambucus	Samb.
Spongia tost	Spong.
Stibium	Stib.
Sulphur	Sulph.
Veratrum alb	Verat. alb.
Veratrum viride	Verat. vir.

Tincture used for External Application: Arnica Mont.

PREFACE.

It has been for a long time the design of the writer, a design seconded by many under his care who were desirous of having such a book in their houses, to prepare a manual of directions, which, with an accompanying case of medicines, might be used in such cases of emergency as are most liable to occur, and in which it is important that some means of relief should be resorted to at once; but until the present time he has been unable to prepare it, though daily more and more convinced of the need of such a work.

Some time may frequently elapse, and this, particularly in the country, before the services of a physician can be obtained, and in the interval, properly directed remedies may be the means not only of alleviating much distress, but often of preserving life.

It is to meet the class of cases above referred to, that this manual has been prepared. The writer has not desired to present a manual of the treatment of diseases generally, partly because the perusal of a single book is not sufficient to render families competent to treat all diseases, and partly because there is at present no lack of works on domestic practice

He has, however, given directions for the management of a few diseases, such as may not be considered of sufficient gravity to demand the assistance of a physician, or such as may occur and require treatment, when there may be no physician accessible, as during absence from the city in the summer. in travelling, &c. Among these are included dysentery, diarrhœa, colds, headaches, sore throats, constipation, colic, &c. Directions are given also for the treatment of sea-sickness, and a short account of the nature and treatment of diphtheria is also given, as its prevalence for the last four or five years makes every one desirous of knowing how the disease may be recognized when it makes its appearance.

The work is divided into four parts: Part I. relating to diseases proper; Part II. to the treatment of cases of poisoning; Part III. to almost every variety of accident, and Part IV. to a resumé of the effects and indications for the use of the various remedies recommended in the work.

The writer has studied carefully throughout the work, to avoid overloading it with unnecessary symptoms, descriptions, and remedies which would require a great deal of time to understand, at a moment when every instant might be precious, but to describe the disease and proper treatment in such a manner, and so concisely, that the disease, the rem edy, and the dose may be recognised as easily as possible, and has given as few remedies as possible, so, in short, that the directions may be of *practical use,* and fulfil the objects for which they are intended.

Under the head of "Poisoning," he has included only those cases liable to occur from the most common poisons, such as are most frequently kept in households, and are most liable to be given by mistake or in overdoses.

Both the diseases and accidents are arranged throughout the book in *alphabetical* order.

This work also differs from all others, in the fact that the directions throughout the book are exclusively for the employment of the *strongest preparations* of Homœopathic medicines in general use; the pellets which are prescribed in other works not being referred to.

For the benefit of those who possess the book, without the case of medicines, it may be stated that the directions are, when liquids are prescribed, for the strong tinctures, and when powders are given, the *first trituration,* except Mercurius Corrosivus, of which the second trituration should be given.

H. B. MILLARD.

7 EAST 27TH STREET,
NEW-YORK. MAY 1ST, 1863

PREFACE TO THE THIRD EDITION.

In presenting to the public the Third edition of this work, I beg to remind the critical reader, that the preparation of a medical work, as small even as this, for the use of others than physicians, is by no means an easy task. The difficulty consists in being obliged to write upon the nature, distinction, and treatment of serious diseases, in a manner perfectly comprehensible to readers presumedly ignorant of medical terms and of everything pertaining to medicine. To write for physicians is much easier, inasmuch as the writer's ideas and descriptions, whether good or bad, are comprehended with facility.

And beside, in order to avoid that great evil—a great book—and to save the reader the labor of studying a dozen pages to ascertain the proper remedy, I am obliged to make difficult things plain in a few lines.

I have endeavored to prepare a book for *use*, not to impress readers by a display of learned terms; and the extensive sale the work has had, induces me to hope that I have to some extent succeeded in my purpose.

Important additions have been made in the present edition, by inserting an Index of Remedies useful in various complaints, rules for the use of several remedies not mentioned in the former editions, and adding chapters on Fevers, Scarlatina, and Measles.

H. B. M.

47 EAST 25TH STREET,
NEW-YORK, JANUARY 1, 1871.

INTRODUCTION.

General Directions and Explanations, Selections of Remedies, Doses, &c.

1.—In the occurrence of any of the diseases or accidents mentioned in this work, send for medical assistance, unless it be in diseases not attended with immediate danger, as headaches, colds, &c., or unless medical assistance is not within reach. Do this, no matter how confident of yourselves; in the meantime, employ the various measures for relief that are directed. The aid of a physician is always desirable, as you might possibly mistake the character of the disease; and there are also, in certain cases, some important remedies and measures which can be employed only by a physician, and which consequently have not been alluded to in this work.

The Selection of Remedies.

2.—Do not think, that because a certain remedy is not recommended for *every* symptom presented by the patient's case, or because the case does not present every symptom given under the remedy, that that remedy is not to be employed. The rule generally is, to select that remedy which seems to be suited to the *greatest number* of the symptoms of the case, or the most important ones, or which is suited to certain causes or conditions.

3.—Sometimes no *single* remedy will be found to cover all the principal conditions and symptoms of the case, but there may be *two* remedies which will be suited to all the symptoms. For instance, in the treatment of certain cases of dysentery (see Dysentery), Mercurius Solubilis and Colocynth; in the treatment of headaches, Nux and Belladona; in the treatment of diarrhœa, Arsenic and Veratrum, or Ipecacuanha and Veratrum may *both* be given in alternation.

4.—Where there is a decidedly feverish condition, Aconite may generally be employed with advantage, whether as one of the regular remedies, or whether given from time to time in conjunction with the other remedies.

Doses and Preparation of the Medicines.

5.—The doses of all the medicines for an adult are as follows (unless where different directions are given under the head of treatment): Each of the tinctures or liquids is to be prepared by mixing five drops with half a tumbler of water. The dose of this is a tea-spoonful.

The tumblers should be perfectly clean, should be kept covered, and a separate tea-spoon used for each tumbler.

The dose of any powder is about five grains (except when a different quantity is directed). It is not necessary that the *exact* weight should be given; this could not be done without weighing it; it will be sufficiently accurate to give as near the quantity mentioned as possible.

Or, the dose of any of the powders for an adult may be set down at about as much as will lie heaped up on an old-fashioned silver three-cent piece; that quantity weighing five or six grains.

To a child from two to four years old, doses about one-half the size of those directed for adults may be given; that is, two and a half grains of a powder; and *two* drops of a tincture may be mixed with *half* a tumbler of water, *of which a tea-spoonful is to be given.* To a child from four to fifteen years old, about three-quarters of an adult dose may be given. The powders, unless directions to the contrary are given, are always to be given dry on the tongue.

DOSES FOR INFANTS.—For an infant between one

and two years, two drops; and for an infant from six months to one year old, one drop may be mixed with half a tumbler of water; and for an infant under six months, a drop with three quarters of a tumbler, of which the dose is a tea-spoonful. The powders are not to be given dry, as to adults. Five or six grains are to be dissolved in a third of a tumbler of water, of which the dose is a tea-spoonful to a child between one and two years old, and half a tea-spoonful to a child less than a year old. The medicines should, in all cases, be thoroughly mixed.

7.—DOSES OF CASTOR OIL.—The dose of Castor Oil for a person over fifteen years of age is two table-spoonfuls; for a child from five to fifteen years old a tablespoonful, though often a larger dose than this will be necessary to act upon the bowels; for a child under two years old, one teaspoonful, though often a second teaspoonful will have to be given.

EMETICS.—Doses of Sulphate of zinc as an emetic. Recourse to this remedy may be necessary in cases of poisoning, and in certain other conditions to be hereafter referred to.

The average dose of Sulphate of Zinc for an adult is fifteen grains. If, however, a poison have been taken, such as opium or laudanum, twenty grains should be given, followed by ten more if vomiting do not take place in seven or eight minutes: to a child from ten to fifteen years old, ten to fifteen grains; to a child five to ten years old, six to ten grains; to a child two to five years old, four to eight grains; to a child from one to two years old, four grains; to a child under one year, two to three grains. Sulphate of zinc should be given dissolved in a little water.

A number of powders of Sulphate of Zinc, of different sizes, accompany the cases of medicines.

9.—FREQUENCY OF DOSES.—No exact rule can be given for this. Where two remedies are given in alternation, it will be necessary to give them more frequently than if only one were given. Where the symptoms are very severe, as in dysentery or diarrhœa, a dose might be given as often as every half hour; or as often in headache, if the pain be very severe. As a general thing, the remedies should be given from every half hour to every two hours. Directions as to the frequency of the doses, have however generally been given under each article.

Finally, rules have been given for the treatment of diseases only ***during the attacks;*** the treatment during the interval has been left for the physician.

As the case accompanying this work contains a number of medicines which are poisonous, except when given in medicinal doses, they should be taken always as nearly as possible in the prescribed doses, and should be carefully kept *out of the reach of children.*

When however you are obliged to treat a case without the assistance of a physician, and you have commenced the use of certain remedies, do not, because the disease does not get better *at once*, change the medicines for fear you are not giving the right ones. Decide upon the proper medicines according to your best judgment, and after using them for a considerable time, if the symptoms are not relieved, you can select other remedies.

Every family in which there are children, should have in the house a syringe. The best and most convenient are the flexible india rubber syringes now in use ; they come supplied with various sized tubes, and can be obtained at most druggists. Davidson's or Richardson's are among the best. They are useful, not only in many diseases of children, but of adults also.

PART I.

THE TREATMENT OF DISEASES.

APOPLEXY.

A fully developed attack of apoplexy is characterized by loss of sensation, thought and voluntary motion, and occurs in one of three ways.

1. The head, neck and face are full and flushed, the breathing deep and puffing, or slow ; the patient lies as if in a deep sleep. This condition may be developed suddenly, or may come on very slowly, the patient sometimes being at first affected with drowsiness, which terminates in insensibility, and in this form of seizure.

2. The attack commences with nausea, vomiting, faintness, or pain in the head, which is generally followed immediately, or an uncertain time after, by stupor.

3. The attack is characterised by loss of power from the very beginning (paralysis), in some part of the body, or by loss of speech.

An attack of apoplexy may be preceded by dizziness, drowsiness, headache, a feeling of fullness in the head, noises in the ear, confusion of ideas, nausea, vomiting, loss of memory, flashes of light, or specks before the eyes

DIAGNOSIS.*—Is is important that this disease should not be mistaken for epilepsy, which it sometimes resembles, as the management of the two diseases is quite different. It may be distinguished from epilepsy by the circumstance, that in apoplexy the breathing is free and unembarrassed, though it may be heavy, while in epilepsy the respiration is very difficult, and is obstructed by the closing of the larynx.† Epilepsy is generally attended with convulsive and spasmodic movements, and there is forcible closure of the jaws. In apoplexy the patient lies senseless or still. An attack of epilepsy is comparatively short, lasting from a few seconds to several minutes, and is succeeded by a heavy sleep. In an epileptic fit too, the face is greatly distorted, the pupils are dilated, and there is frothing at the mouth.

TREATMENT.—Loosen all articles of clothing about the chest and throat which may interfere with respi-

---

* "Diagnosis." This word, one frequently used in describing diseases, signifies the recognition or distinguishing a disease from any other, for which it might be mistaken.

† "Larynx." The projection felt on the front of the throat and under the jaw. It feels like a knob or hard ball. It is commonly called "Adam's apple." It forms the upper extremity of the windpipe, and contains the vocal organs.

ration; raise the patient up, with the head elevated, and give an injection of five or six teaspoonfuls of spirits of turpentine beaten up with the yolk of an egg and mixed with a pint of water; if the turpentine be not at hand, give an injection of warm water.

In the first variety, apply cloths wet with cold water to the head, and as soon as the patient can swallow, give *Ac.* and *Bell.* in alternation every fifteen minutes, till the symptoms are alleviated, when they may be given half an hour apart.

If the attack be accompanied by full face, heavy breathing, *stupor*, great drowsiness, slow, full pulse and moaning, give *Bell.* and *Opium* in the same manner.

If the attack seem to be of the second variety, and there be dizziness, nausea, paleness, drowsiness, confusion of ideas and pain, give *Ac.* and *Nux*, in the same manner. *Nux* is peculiarly applicable, if the patient be dyspeptic, or is accustomed to the use of ardent spirits.

When an attack seems to be setting in, and there are fulness of the head, redness of the face and eyes, headache, dizziness, and general symptoms of congestion of the head, give *Ac.* and *Bell.* in alternation, from fifteen minutes to an hour apart, according to the severity of the symptoms.

If there are fulness, pain, *nausea*, dizziness, and

there exist disorders of the stomach, bowels or liver, give *Ac.* and *Nux.* at similar intervals.

ABOVE ALL, when an attack is threatened or has set in, bear in mind this one rule: *Always produce an evacuation of the bowels.* If the attack is setting in and the symptoms are not severe, this may be done by the administration of a full dose of castor oil. If the attack have set in, or the symptoms are severe, resort to injections of warm water, or, what is better, turpentine prepared as directed above.

When the attack is fully developed, it is only in the first variety that much good can be expected from immediate medication; in this, however, the danger may be often totally averted by the remedies. Attacks of the other two varieties may also often be prevented by them, if they are administered as soon as the symptoms are observed.

Note. An overloaded stomach, as after an immoderate dinner, may be sometimes followed by symptoms of apoplexy; the patient falling down, the head becoming flushed and turgid, and the breathing labored. Where the stomach is known to be overloaded, elevate the head, give an emetic (twenty grains of Sulphate of Zinc) in a little water, and produce an evacuation from the bowels.

II.

Bleeding from the Lungs,

Is often preceded by some oppression of the chest, or by a slight cough. The blood is of a *bright red* color, and has a saltish taste ; it is generally brought up in mouthfuls, or in small quantities at a time ; the quantity raised may vary from a teaspoonful to cupfuls.

TREATMENT.—If it be slight, no immediate treatment is necessary ; if it be at all profuse, place the patient in a recumbent position, with the head raised, permit a free circulation of air, give cold drinks, and apply cloths wet with cold water to the chest. Internally, salt and water may be given. *Do not be alarmed, as the immediate consequences of hæmoptysis† are seldom fatal.

III.

Bleeding from the Nose.

If bleeding from the nose occur in a robust, plethoric person, or in a person who is subject to it, or who is subject to rush of blood to the head, giddiness and headache, or if it occur in a female, in place of the regular monthly sickness, or if it take the place of bleeding from piles, it is generally salutary, *and should not be arrested unless it continue a long time,* or threaten to produce exhaustion. When thus profuse, or when it produces exhaustion, or when it oc-

* Hamamelis, five drops at a dose, in alternation with Aconite, half an hour to an hour apart, will be found very useful.

† Hæmoptysis, Bleeding from the Lungs.

curs in weakly, pale individuals, or is the result of an injury, a blow, &c., measures should be resorted to to suppress it.

Treatment.—The patient should *sit up*, keep perfectly quiet, and stimulants should be avoided; then the most convenient and effectual measures that can be resorted to by non-medical persons are as follows:

1. Raise and hold perpendicularly above the head, the arm of the side from which the blood flows, and with the other hand close firmly the bleeding nostril; this will generally stop an ordinary nose bleed.

2. If necessary, apply cloths wet with cold water to the forehead, nose and back of the neck, or a piece of cold metal may be applied to the back of the neck. Employ these measures perseveringly. If the bleeding do not then cease,

3. Press into the nostril bunches of clean cotton wool (cotton batting) until it is filled as full as possible.

Catarrhs, Colds, Coughs, Sore Throat.

In prescribing the treatment of these affections, only a few general remedies have been recommended, adapted to the most common symptoms which these disorders give rise to. No other class of affections is accompanied by a greater variety of symptoms, or demands a greater variety of remedies, or a more thorough knowledge of their character. Their *de-*

tailed treatment has therefore not been entered upon, as to have done this would not only have required a good deal of space, but would have been foreign to the object of the directions, which are intended simply as guides in cases of emergency, and in the treatment of ordinary affections, where no physician is at hand.

For ordinary cold affecting the system generally, with or without chillness and heat, pains in the limbs, lassitude, feverishness or headache, *Aconite* and *Stibium* should be given in alternation two hours apart.

DOSE, ETC.—For an adult, six drops of *Aconite*, to be mixed with half a tumbler of water, of which the dose is a teaspoonful. The dose of *Stibium* is as much as will lie on a three cent piece, heaped up.

For colds accompanied by severe pain in and about the eyes, root of the nose, and forehead, give *Ars.* and *Stib.* in alternation, two hours apart.

DOSE.—Of *Stibium*, the same as above; the *Arsenicum* to be prepared by mixing four drops with half a glass of water; dose, a teaspoonful.

For cold affecting principally the chest or windpipe, and accompanied by *soreness* or *tenderness*, give *Stibium* and *Merc. Sol.* in alternation, two hours apart.

DOSE.—As much of each as will lie on a three cent piece heaped up.

For cold affecting principally the chest or windpipe, and accompanied by considerable accumulation of phlegm in the throat, *Stibium* and *Hepar* are the proper remedies.

DOSE.—Same as in paragraph above.

If the cold be accompanied by pain in the chest, tightness and oppression and aching, with short, quick breathing, give *Stib.* and *Phos.* in alternation, an hour or two apart.

DOSE.—Add four drops of *Phos.* to half a tumbler of water, and give a teaspoonful at a dose. The dose of *Stibium* for an adult is about five grains, to be taken dry on the tongue. For an infant or child, one to three drops of *Phos.* may be added to half a tumbler of water; and for an infant, about ten grains of *Stibium* may be dissolved in half a tumbler of water, and a teaspoonful given at a dose. For a child from two to five years old, two or three grains of *Stibium* may be given at a dose, and three drops of *Phos.* may be mixed in half a tumbler of water, of which a teaspoonful is to be given. Care should always be taken not to give *Stibium* in over doses, as even the Homœopathic preparations sometimes produce vomiting.

For hard dry cough, *Stibium* and *Nux.* should be given in alternation, two hours apart.

DOSE.—As much *Stibium* to be taken at a dose as

will lie on a three cent piece. The *Nux.* to be prepared by mixing five drops in half a glass of water; dose a teaspoonful.

For hard dry cough, accompanied with *soreness*, give *Merc. Dulc.* and *Stib.* in alternation, two hours apart.

DOSE.—As much of each as will lie on a three cent piece.

For a hard, loose, rattling cough, particularly if worse night and morning, or if accompanied by a cold in the head, give ***Kali Bich.*** and ***Stibium*** in alternation, two hours apart.

DOSES.—Same as above. Each dose of the *Kali* to be dissolved in a little water.

Colds affecting the Throat—Sore Throat.

For sore throat, accompanied by bright redness of the throat, aching pain, and difficulty of swallowing, *Bell.* and *Merc. Sol.* should be given in alternation, two hours apart.

DOSE.—Each of these medicines to be prepared by mixing five drops with half a glass of water. A teaspoonful to be given at a dose.

For sore throat, accompanied by soreness, difficulty of swallowing, ulceration and accumulation of phlegm in the throat, give *Merc. Protiod.* and *Stib.* two hours apart.

Dose.—Five grains of each of these medicines at a dose; to a child above two years of age, half these doses.

If there be *hoarseness* or *soreness* in the larynx or windpipe, give *Spong.* and *Stib.* two hours apart.

Dose.—Five drops of Spongia to be mixed with half a tumbler of water; a teaspoonful to be given at a dose. Five grains of Stibium at a dose.

Catarrhal Affections in Infants.

Upon infants these troubles make a much more profound impression than upon adults, and should be carefully attended to.

Among the most important and common affections of this kind to which they are subject, are

1. *Cold in the head.*

When accompanied by sneezing, running at the nose, watery eyes, and a stuffed up condition of the nostrils, known as "snuffles," the child being unable to breathe through the nose, give *Stib.* and *Nux.* in alternation, one hour apart.

Dose.—Five or six grains of *Stibium* may be dissolved in half a tumbler of water, and two drops of *Nux* added to a similar quantity. A tea-spoonful to be given at a dose.

2. In colds of infants, accompanied by fever, rapid or difficult breathing, give *Verat. Vir.* and

Kali Hyd. in alternation, from half an hour to an hour apart; or, if the breathing become very rapid, as often as half an hour apart, until there is an improvement.

DOSES.—The *Verat Vir.* and *Kali* to be prepared according to directions for doses on pages IX and X.

3. If the cold be accompanied by hard, dry cough, give *Stib.* and *Nux* in alternation, two hours apart.

DOSE.—Same as in case 11.

If accompanied by a loose, rattling cough, or by a rattling of phlegm in the chest, as if it were loaded with phlegm, give *Verat. Vir.* and *Merc. Cor.* in alternation, an hour and a half or two hours apart. If there be fever, or the respiration be hurried, *Verat. Vir.* and *Merc. Sol.* must be given.

DOSE.—The liquids to be prepared as in case 1. About four grains of *Merc. Sol.* to be given at a dose.

Colic.

SYMPTOMS.—Violent pains in the abdomen, generally coming on in paroxysms; the bowels usually confined; sometimes nausea and vomiting. The pains are aching, cutting, pressing or tearing; sometimes so violent as to cause the sufferer to writhe about the bed or floor in agony. The pain is generally not increased, but relieved by *firm* pressure.

Causes.—Among the most common are cold; moisture ; a chill ; unripe or indigestible food. Sometimes, obstructions of the intestines.

TREATMENT.—If unaccompanied by inflammation, which may be recognized by the pain being *greatly increased* by gentle or hard pressure, try at once to get the bowels to move by giving a dose of castor oil. The dose for an adult is two full tablespoons; for a child from five to ten years old, half that quantity; if this do not produce an evacuation from the bowels in an hour or two, put patient in a warm bath, and while in, give copious injections of warm water. The temperature of the bath should be quite high, and the patient should be allowed to remain in ten or fifteen minutes. Great alleviation of the pain will be obtained by applying flannels wrung out in hot water to the abdomen.

The medicines to be taken internally are as follows:

I. If there is great flatulence or distension of the bowels by wind, if the colic proceed from cold, give *Mercurius Dulcis* and *Nux. Vom.* in alternation, from half an hour to an hour apart, lessening the doses in frequency, in proportion as the pains become less frequent or less severe.

II. If the pains are low down in the bowels, pinching, griping, cutting or bearing down, particularly if accompanied by cramps or pains in the legs, give *Merc. Dulc.* and *Coloc.* at the same intervals as in the preceding case.

III. If the pains are principally about the navel, give *Merc. Dulc.* and *Bell.* unless *Nux.* should be indicated, as in case I.

Doses, Administration, &c.—The dose of *Merc. Dulc.* in a ***severe*** case of colic, should be about six grains. Four drops of *Coloc.* or five of *Nux.* or *Bell*, is to be mixed with half a tumbler of water; the dose of either of these is a teaspoonful.

The intervals of the administration of the doses must vary according to the severity of the pain, and must be greater as the pains become less. They may be given from the beginning, half an hour to two hours apart. Sometimes a single dose of each, with the other means directed, will make the patient comfortable.

Colic of Infants.

Infants at the breast are particularly subject to colicky pains and accumulation of wind in the intestines. These pains are characterized by a variety of symptoms. The child cries violently, draw its legs upon its belly or twists about; the abdomen feels bloated; the crying may be so violent as to cause the face to turn purple, and the child appears as if it were on the point of going into spasms.

Causes.—Frequently the disorder proceeds from a cold; it may be caused by a confined state of the bowels; by irritating properties of the mother's milk;

by unsuitable or impure food; by improper food, cabbage, pork, etc., eaten by the mother or nurse.

Treatment.—If the bowels are confined, a movement should be produced by giving an injection of warm water.

If the bowels are inclined to costiveness; if the passages are *not* too loose and are not like diarrhœa, if the passages are healthy, give *Coloc.* and *Nux.*

If, with the colicky pains, there is *looseness* of the bowels, the passages being either too frequent, or thin, or unnatural in their appearance, *Coloc.* and *Rheum* may be given; if the colic proceed from cold, *Jalap* may be substituted for the *Rheum*, (see also "Diarrhœa"). In case the attack be very severe, additional relief will be obtained by the application all over the bowels of a piece of flannel wrung out of hot water, and applied as warm as it can be borne. This should be covered with dry flannel, in order that chilliness or cold may not be produced. The wet flannel may be changed every half hour, until relief is obtained. When there is much flatulence, bloating of the abdomen, &c., the bowels may be rubbed diligently for a little while with warm sweet oil. This may be done frequently every day with advantage, when there is a tendency to colicky pains.

Dose, Administration, &c.—For an infant under a year old, two drops of either of the remedies mentioned above may be added to a glass of water, and the two remedies selected may be given while the paroxysm is *very distressing*, in alternation, fifteen minutes apart, until one or two doses of each have been given; after that, if the pain continue very severe, every half hour in turn, until relief is obtained. After that, if the child do not sleep; if the crying and pain continue to be somewhat troublesome, they may be given an hour or two apart. The medicines and the other means recommended will generally be found to relieve all ordinary cases of colic in infants. In case relief were not produced by any of these measures, a warm bath might be given. It will seldom, however, be necessary.

It is a common custom for nurses and mothers, in their impatience and anxiety to quiet the child, to give it gin, &c. It is better not to do this; and by no means be tempted to give any of the innumerable anodynes, cordials and soothing syrups which are in such general use. It is little less than inhuman to administer quack medicines to infants.

The "soothing" principle of nearly all these preparations is opium, (a remedy which even medical men give to infants with great caution). Syrup of poppies and paragoric are objectionable for the same reason. There are numerous instances on record in which coroners' inquests have disclosed the fact that children have lost their lives from the use of these various preparations, and it is no exaggeration to say that they have shortened the lives of thousands of infants. Peppermint, aniseed tea, are frequently not objectionable, when the passages are perfectly healthy, and there is *no diarrhœa*. The other remedies however, will be almost always found much more satisfactory.

Constipation of Infants.

Constipation in infants may be attended with the most disastrous results. Where it is habitual, a physician will of course be consulted. When it is necessary to produce a movement of the bowels, an injection of warm water may be given, or a piece of soap may be shaped like the finger, introduced into the bowel, and allowed to remain there a few moments. When it is not necessary that an immediate evacuation of the bowels should be produced, *Nux* and *Sulphur* may be given in alternation, two hours apart, until the bowels move.

Dose.—For a child less than a year old, the dose of Sulphur is as much as can be heaped up on a three cent piece. The Nux is to be prepared by mixing two drops with two-thirds of a glass of water, of which the dose is a teaspoonful. For a child over a year old, half as much again Sulphur may be given and three drops of Nux, mixed with a glass of water.

Convulsions of Children.

While convulsions constitute a class of diseases the most alarming to which children are liable, on the other hand it is no slight gratification to know, that in a large proportion of cases, properly selected and applied remedies will afford speedy relief. When a child is seized with convulsions, bear in mind these two important points.

1. Be self-possessed and composed. Do not send every one in different directions, for every remedy which suggests itself. In this, as in all other cases of sudden and great danger, self-possession, and ability to consider what the matter is and what should be done, is of more use than can be easily imagined.

2. Ascertain as nearly as possible, to which of the causes to be hereafter mentioned the convulsion is owing. These two points observed, you can consider the case rationally and with a basis on which to select the remedies.

The most common causes of convulsions are:

1. The irritation of teething.

2. The sudden suppression of diarrhœa which often attends teething.

3. Irritating or indigestible food; unripe fruit.

cake, confectionary, &c. Even a bit of orange peel may produce them.

4. Constipation.

5. Flatulence.

6. Worms. Do not however, attribute the convulsion to this cause, unless you are certain of the presence of worms by the child's having passed them. This is the only reliable evidence of their existence.

7. The sudden disappearance of eruptions, as in scarlet fever or measles; the imperfect development of the eruption in these diseases; the sudden suppression of skin diseases, ulcers, scald head, &c.

8. Irritating properties of the mother's milk.

9. There are numerous other causes, less frequent, however, or more obscure, as blows; falls; water on the brain; inflammation of the brain; fright; cold. Sometimes, indeed, it is impossible to assign a *direct* cause for them, and they appear to be owing to extreme sensitiveness of the intestinal canal, brain and nervous system.

In the first year of life the brain is very imperfectly developed, while that part of the nervous system which regulates digestion and nutrition, predominates in its influence upon the system, over the brain. The digestive system working with so great activity at this time, and the brain with so little, the child being nothing more or less than a young growing animal.

and this system being so liable to derangement convulsions are much more liable to occur at this period than at any other. After the first year the mortality from convulsions diminishes rapidly. It is important, therefore, that the greatest care should be exercised at this time of life, in everything that affects the digestive system of the child; the state of the bowels, the process of teething, etc.

SYMPTOMS.—There is no mistaking a convulsion when it has once set in. It may come on suddenly or be preceded by constipation, sudden and violent starting in the sleep, rolling of the eyes, twitching of the fingers, restlessness, oppressed breathing, etc. When any of these symptoms are observed, the child should be carefully watched and remedies corresponding to any cause which may be known to exist, administered.

TREATMENT.—General Indications.

1. Send for a physician.

2. In convulsions from *whatever* cause, proceed at once to produce a movement in the bowels. If the child can *swallow*, and particularly if the trouble be owing to improper food, flatulence, or constipation, give a teaspoonful of castor oil (this dose to a child less than a year old. Beyond that age, a larger dose should be given). An injection may be given in all cases, at the same time, of equal parts of warm

water and milk; of sweet oil and milk; of molasses and water, or of soap and water.

3. If the convulsion be attended with flushed face, fullness of the head, and the child is of a full habit, apply cloths wet with cold water to the head.

4. Give a warm bath; as warm as it can well be borne. Immerse the child all over, and let it remain in the bath five or ten minutes unless the paroxysm begin to abate sooner, when it should be taken out and wrapped in warm blankets; should the paroxysm return, the immersion should be repeated at the expiration of a few minutes.

5. It may not always be necessary to resort to *all* the above remedies; a movement from the bowels, however, should always be produced. In the cases in which an emetic is directed, castor oil should not be given, but an injection should be resorted to. Sometimes the movement of the bowels will end the convulsion at once; sometimes the convulsion may be so slight as to render it unnecessary to employ the warm bath.

6. If a physician can be obtained in a short time, do not resort to the remedies mentioned below, but leave them till his arrival. If, however, medical assistance be not at hand, or cannot be employed within a reasonable time, employ the various remedies according to the following indications.

The following special remedies should be given not so much with reference to the nature of the convulsion, as to the *cause*, when the latter is known.

1. If the child's stomach is known to have been overloaded with unsuitable food, pastry, nuts, raisins, etc., give an *emetic*, recourse to this means of relief being in some cases indispensable. For mode of administering the emetic, dose, etc., see Introduction page XI.

2. If the convulsion be owing to suppressed eruption in skin diseases, add a couple of tablespoonfuls of mustard to the bath, and if the eruption be that of measles, give, if the child can swallow, *Bry.* every half hour; if the convulsion be owing to the suppressed or imperfect eruption of scarlet fever, give *Bell.* at the same intervals.

DOSES, ETC.—Each of the two remedies mentioned above is to be prepared by mixing two drops with two-thirds of a tumbler of water and giving a teaspoonful at a dose. A dose should be given about every half hour; after two or three doses have been given, or the symptoms have abated, once an hour or once in two hours will be sufficient.

3. If the child is *known* to have worms, *Merc. Dulc.* may be given every three quarters of an hour.

DOSE.—To a child less than two years old, five grains mixed with a little white sugar; more than two years, five to eight grains. This medicine may be discontinued as soon as it has been followed by green stools, or by the passage of worms.

GENERAL REMEDIES,

Suited to the various characteristics of the convulsion, and without particular reference to the cause.

When the child is of a full habit, the pupils are enlarged; there is short, panting, or heavy breathing with oppression of the chest; the child starts while sleeping; the child cries violently; the body becomes stiffly convulsed; the forehead and hands are dry and burning; the face *is red or bloated;* there is redness all over; the eyeballs and features are distorted, give ***Bell.***

DOSE, ETC.—Two drops in two-thirds of a tumbler of water; a teaspoonful from every half hour to every hour.

When there is pale face, twitching of the limbs, spasms or rigidity of the limbs, bending of the head or body backwards, violent shrieks, give *Nux.* This remedy is particularly of value if there be flatulence, colicky pains, constipation, or if the convulsion be caused by any other derangement of the stomach or bowels.

Dose.—The same as in the preceding case.

When there is rolling of the head, twitching of the face, twitching of the legs, dilated, staring pupils, foaming at the mouth, shrieking, pale or fiery red face, give *Hyos.* in the same manner as the medicines in the preceding cases.

When there is lethargy, tremor, heaviness, stupor; heavy breathing; tossing of the arms and legs about; give *Opium.*

Dose.—Same as in the preceding cases.

In convulsions which cannot be traced to a direct cause, but which seem owing to an unnatural irritability of the nervous system, in convulsions which are caused by fright, or are habitual, *Ignatia* is an invaluable remedy. The symptoms to which it is particularly applicable, are violent screaming, tremor, terror; the child wakes from its sleep, uttering piercing cries.

Croup.

Genuine croup is a fever, accompanied by inflammation of the lining membrane of the larynx* and windpipe. In severe or fatal cases, a membrane is formed which covers these parts, the membrane varying in thickness from a thin film to that of wash leather. Sometimes, instead of a membrane, there exist only swelling and redness of the interior of

* *Larynx.* See page 15. note

the larynx and windpipe, or they are covered with a thick fluid.

Croup is an exceedingly rare disease in infants less than a year old. It occurs most frequently during the second year; after that, generally between the second and seventh years. Fat children are most subject to it, and it comes on in most cases in the night.

The causes of croup are those of ordinary colds or catarrh; sudden exposure, even a draught from an open door, may produce it.

Symptoms preceding an attack of Croup.—An attack of croup may come on suddenly, but is commonly preceded by certain symptoms by which its approach may be foretold. The principal of these are the various symptoms of a cold, which are always to be regarded with suspicion if they are accompanied by *hoarseness* or *huskiness*, or by a rough, *hoarse* cough. Catarrhal symptoms do not often indicate croup unless accompanied by some degree of hoarseness. Together with these symptoms, the child may be feverish, restless, dull or drowsy. These symptoms may be followed by croup a short time after their appearance, though perhaps not for several days.

SYMPTOMS OF CROUP.—Dry, hoarse, husky cough, often very violent; hoarse voice, with a sound like the crowing of a cock; this hoarseness of the voice is one of the most characteristic signs of croup; sometimes complete loss of voice; difficulty of breathing; crowing inspiration, becoming long and wheezing as the attack continues; fever; hot, flushed face; when the cough is severe or long, the child seems almost on the point of suffocation. In severe cases, as the disease advances, the voice becomes almost or quite extinct; the child stretches back its neck; the eyes are protruded; the face becomes discolored or pale, and the little sufferer looks as if dying from suffocation.

When the attack comes on suddenly, the child is roused from sleep by paroxysms of hoarse or rattling cough which almost threaten to suffocate it, or with panting, wheezing, difficult respiration, with fever. The symptoms may subside entirely and the child appear perfectly well, though some hoarseness and fever may remain; the paroxysms are liable however to return and become more frequent. An attack of croup, though subdued one night, is liable to make its appearance several nights in succession.

The above constitute the symptoms of a fully developed case of croup. Some of these may be hardly perceptible, and all may be less violent than is here represented, and there will also be modifications of them. There will however be but little difficulty in recognizing the disease from this description.

TREATMENT.—1. Wrap a piece of flannel, folded and wet in cold water, around the child's throat, and cover this with a *dry* flannel.

2. Dissolve one of the one grain powders of *Tartar Emetic* in a tumbler of warm water, and give a teaspoonful every five minutes; as symptoms of nausea appear, diminish the frequency of the dose, giving it every ten or fifteen minutes; the medicine should be given so as to keep the child just on the point of nausea, or nauseated as much as he can be without vomiting. *Do not vomit the child*, this will only exhaust it, and do the disease itself no good.

3. If the attack be accompanied by decided febrile symptoms, or fever, give *Aconite* every ten or twenty minutes, between the Tartar Emetic, according to its severity. It may be prepared by mixing four drops with half a tumbler of water, of which a teaspoonful may be given at a dose.

4. If the child's bowels have not moved within a reasonable time, give an injection of warm water, or milk, or molasses and water.

5. If the attack be severe and *obstinate*, a warm bath should be prepared, as warm as it can be comfortably borne. The child should remain in the bath at least ten minutes, and should then be wiped dry, enveloped in warm blankets, and put to bed.

6. After the violence of the paroxysm is subdued.

give the *Ac.* and *Tart. Emet.* at intervals of from half an hour to two hours apart, according to the amount of hoarseness, cough, fever, &c., remaining.

7. But if the breathing become free; and as the cough becomes free and loose, the voice more distinct, and particularly if there seem to be an accumulation of phlegm and a rattling in the throat, give *Tart. Emet.* and *Hepar* at intervals of from half an hour to two hours apart. The dose of Hepar for an infant is two or three grains.

False Croup, Spasmodic Croup, Child Crowing, Millar's Asthma, &c.

CAUSES--NATURE, &c.—This disease, known by all the above names, is scarcely less dangerous than, and resembles, in many of its symptoms, genuine croup. Unlike croup, however, it occurs most frequently during the first year, or during the period of teething. It consists in a spasm of the muscles of the larynx,* by which the aperture through which the air is admitted into the windpipe is narrowed or closed entirely. When occurring during the period of teething, it is generally produced by the irritation set up by that process, or by some of the irregularities so frequently attendant upon it, as diarrhœa, flatulence, constipation, catarrh, &c.

* Larynx. For definition, see page 15.

It may also occur before or after dentition, and is generally owing to some of the causes calculated to produce convulsions, as enumerated in the chapter on convulsions.

SYMPTOMS.—The child is seized suddenly, generally in the night, with difficulty of breathing; it throws up its arms, and makes the most violent exertions to get breath, but it seems impossible for the air to enter; the child struggles violently; the face becomes pale and a cold sweat breaks out upon the forehead. The stoppage of breath may last for a few seconds to one or two minutes, and the attack at length terminates by the child taking a long, full breath, generally shrill or crowing. This is the most favorable termination of the attack, and breathing then goes on regularly.

Sometimes, however, though not commonly, the attack may be so severe as to become a real convulsion, the thumbs being drawn in, the hands clenched, the feet turned in upon the ancle, the body bent backwards, and the face distorted and pale.

The attack may occur in the day-time; often being so slight as to render treatment unnecessary, and may be produced by a fit of crying or anger, or it may come on while the child is nursing, sometimes amounting to no more than a short stoppage of breath, or a slight *crowing* sound may be heard with the child's inspiration. Sometimes even during these slight attacks, the thumb will be closed, the fingers drawn tightly in, or the great toe drawn a little apart from the others. These paroxysms, however, if not checked, are liable to become more frequent, and increase, till they equal in severity the attacks described above.

Between the paroxysms, the breathing is in no wise obstructed.

Symptoms preceding an Attack.—Sometimes the attack is not heralded by any pre-existing symptoms. Oftener, however, the child does not enjoy perfect health before the attack, nor does it often attack children whose health is perfectly good. It seems drooping, peevish, restless; its bowels may be confined, or it may be suffering from diarrhœa, or from teething. If the attacks occur frequently, it remains more or less out of health; during the intervals, the breathing is anxious, the child restless, or starts from sleep in affright.

Treatment.—During the paroxysm—

1. Sprinkle cold water on the face.
2. Apply to the throat a flannel wet with water as *warm* as it can be borne.
3. If the warm bath can be prepared without too much delay, employ it, immersing the legs and lower part of the body.

4. Give an injection of warm water or of milk and water.

5. If the spasm be not accompanied with catarrh, let the wind blow freely over the face and chest; *not, however, on the back.*

6. Do not attempt to force medicines down the throat while the child is choking, but as soon as the child can *swallow*, give *Samb.* every half hour until complete relief is obtained.

DOSE.—As much as will lie on a three cent piece, not heaped up.

As the paroxysms are liable to return after they have once made their appearance, see that all exciting causes of this complaint, as constipation, worms, improper food, swollen gums, &c., are removed. The intermediate treatment, however, should be left to the physician.

Distinguishing Marks of "Child Crowing," or "Spasmodic Croup," and Croup.

The only disease for which there is any danger of mistaking this affection is croup. It is, however, of the utmost importance, that the two diseases should not be mistaken for each other, as their nature and treatment are entirely different. They may be generally recognized without much difficulty, by the description of each disease given above. Additional and *certain* marks of distinction are the following:

In "Child Crowing," the attacks come on suddenly, without generally being preceded by any but slight symptoms; the spasm lasts but a short time, and the breathing is *perfectly free in the intervals*; there is no fever, and seldom any cough; the voice rarely becomes extinct; additional evidence of "Child Crowing" is that it is generally owing to some of the causes of nervous irritation mentioned above.

Croup is generally preceded by decided catarrhal symptoms and hoarseness; there is more or less fever, which *continues between* the paroxysms; the breathing is not free *between* the paroxysms, and the voice remains hoarse; the voice becomes muffled or wholly extinct; the cough has more of a brassy, husky character, though the crowing inspiration is much alike in the two diseases; and above all, almost always comes on *after* the first year of age.

Diarrhœa of Grown Persons and Children.

The cause of the diarrhœa should be ascertained, if possible, and the remedies selected with reference to it. Some exciting cause will generally be found. Among the most common are indigestible food, unripe fruit, sudden suppression of perspiration, a chill, a late supper, heat, teething.

Treatment.—If the diarrhœa be caused by undigested food, and there is reason to believe that the bowels are irritated by it, commence the treatment with a dose of castor oil.

1. In diarrhœa caused by cold, a chill, or suppressed perspiration, with thin and watery or dark yellow, or slimy stools, without much constitutional disturbance, with or without slight colicky pains in the bowels, give *Ipecac.* and *Verat. Alb.* in alternation, two hours apart.

DOSE.—For an adult, 5 drops of each of these medicines to be mixed with half a glass of water; for a child from 3 to 15 years of age, four drops, and from 2 to 5 years, three drops with two thirds of a glass of water. Give the two medicines in alternation, half an hour to two hours apart, a teaspoonful to be given at a dose; giving them however as often as every half hour, only when the passages are very frequent; as often, for instance, as every ten or fifteen minutes.

2. If the stools are watery, white or yellow, whether the evacuations are painless or are accompanied by crampy pains in the stomach or bowels, or prostration, give *Arsenicum* and *Verat. Alb.*, the same way and in the same doses as *Ipecac.* and *Verat.* are directed in the paragraph above.

3. When the stools are watery, yellow, slimy, greenish or brownish, dark colored, with or without burning in the stomach, *vomiting*, *nausea*, frequent

desire to drink ; the diarrhœa being worse after eating or drinking, or being produced by eating unripe fruit, give *Arsenicum* and *Veratrum*, in the same doses and in the same manner as *Ipecac.* and *Verat.* are directed in the first paragraph above

4. For dark colored, slimy or mucous, jelly-like stools ; for greenish stools streaked with blood ; greenish stools without blood ; putrid, sour smelling stools ; with or without bearing down behind ; with chilliness, shivering, soreness in the abdomen ; white coated tongue ; stools, with or without cutting pain, give *Merc. Sol.*

DOSE.—For an adult, as much as will lie heaped up on a three cent piece ; to a child 5 to 10 years old, about two thirds, and to a child from 2 to 5 years old, about half that quantity.

5. When there are violent pressing pains in the back, emission of wind from the bowels, *severe* cutting or cramp pains in the bowels, watery passages, and particularly if there are cramps in the legs or arms, give *Colocynth* and *Arsenicum* in the same manner and dose, as the medicines directed under the first verse of " diarrhœa." Watery stools, cramps in the extremities with vomiting, constitute the disease known as Cholera Morbus. These two remedies (Arsenicum and Colocynth) are almost a certain cure for it.

DIET.—The diet in a case of diarrhœa, should be mild and unirritating; solid food should generally be avoided; milk, arrow root, gruel, toast and tea, farina, etc., should be given. This kind of diet, and total abstinence from solid food will cure some cases of diarrhœa.

Diarrhœa of Infants.

"A young infant should have from three to six motions in the twenty-four hours; the color should be of a bright yellow, inclining to orange and the consistence that of thick gruel, and nearly, if not entirely devoid of smell. If the infant instead of having from three to six motions, have more than that number; if they be more watery; if they become slimy and green, or green and in part curdled, and if they have an unpleasant smell, then the child may be said to have diarrhœa."—*Chavasse.*

There is a looseness of the bowels however, which often makes its appearance while the child is teething. It should not be checked, unless it become too frequent or profuse, or exhaustion is produced. The diarrhœa at this time is frequently an effort of nature to relieve the irritation of the nervous system produced by the process of teething. A sudden suppression of it, may lead to trouble of the brain, or to convulsions.

TREATMENT.—In the diarrhœa of infants, the same

remedies are employed, and for the same symptoms as in diarrhœa occurring in adults. When therefore, the diarrhœa of the infant resembles any of the forms described in the preceeding verses on the treatment of diarrhœa, the remedies directed *for* that form may be given.

In addition to these remedies, however, there are others which are particularly applicable to the diarrhœa of infants. These remedies, and the indications for their use, are as follows:

1. In diarrhœa, with watery, slimy, frothy, fermented looking motions, accompanied by flatulence, colicky pain, peevishness, restlessness, screaming; in diarrhœa, proceeding from cold, teething, indigestible food, give *Chamomilla* and *Rheum.*

2. When the stools are thin or slimy, have a fermented appearance, a sour smell, a brownish or grayish color, and particularly if they are accompanied by colic, constant hard crying, screaming, restlesssness; the crying and pains coming on in paroxysms give *Colocynth* and *Rheum.*

3. When the passages are thin and watery, and there is violent screaming, restlessness, crying, &c., *and the attack is thought to proceed from cold, Colocynth* and *Jalap* may be given instead of Colocynth and Rheum.

Whenever the pains, screaming, restlessness, are

very severe, and show no signs of yielding, after several doses have have been administered, a flannel wrung out of hot water, may be applied as directed on page 27.

Doses.—For a child from six months to a year old, two drops of any of the remedies directed for diarrhœa, are to be mixed with a tumbler *full* of water and thoroughly stirred up. For an infant less than six months old, *one* drop to be prepared with three-quarters of a glass of water. When Arsenicum is given to an infant less than six months old, one drop is to be mixed with a *tumbler* of water. When *Mercurius* is given, for a child from six months to a year old, thrice as much as will lie on a three cent piece, heaped up, may be mixed with a tumbler full of water, and to an infant less than six months old half that quantity, with three quarters of a glass of water. The dose of all the medicines thus prepared is a teaspoonfull.

Frequency of Doses.—Unless the passages are *very* frequent, no two medicines need be given oftener than two hours apart, in alternation. If the passages should be very frequent, they may be given from an hour to an hour and a half apart. When however, there is *severe colicky pain*, crying, restlessness, &c., &c., they may be given as often as every half hour apart, until relief is obtained, after that gradually diminishing the frequency of the doses. Where a single medicine only is given, it may be administered every one, two, or three hours.

Diphtheria.

For a disease so formidable in its nature, as this, and so frequently baffling even medical skill, it would be wrong to prescribe, unless for the use of physicians, any plan of treatment. A great variety of means, according to the various symptoms which exist or which may arise, may be required, and for the selection and administration of which, the judgment of a physician is indispensable. A description of this affection is given a place here, in order that the disease may be recognized and receive timely treatment; a few rules as regards its general treatment are given, and directions given for the use of one or two remedies which are frequently of the greatest value in this disease, and which may be resorted to,when a physician cannot be obtained for some time.

Diphtheria is a disease of which the distinguishing characteristic is the formation of a membrane in the throat. It is accompanied by more or less fever.

Symptoms, etc. There is difficulty of swallowing, soreness and pain in the throat, fever, prostration of strength. When the throat is examined, it looks red and inflamed, or, if any membrane have formed, it will be seen situated on the back part of the throat or on the tonsils. Both the amount and the appearance of the membrane vary greatly. Sometimes it is so thin as to resemble a whitish film; sometimes it is as thick as tissue paper, and in the worst forms and in advanced stages, it may become as thick as morocco; its color varies from whitish-grey to a yellowish tinge. Sometimes there may be only one or two small patches, not so large as a split pea, situated perhaps only on one side of the throat; sometimes it will be seen to cover the whole of the tonsils, and the back part of the throat, The above mentioned symptoms are the ones which generally exist; there are others which it is unnecessary to mention here, as sufficient have been given, at least to lead to the suspicion of the existence of diphtheria when these symptoms appear, and to prompt the summoning of medical aid. The diagnosis of this disease, except by a physician, is extremely difficult and uncertain, inasmuch as there are several kinds of sore throat, which are characterized by the symptoms which have been mentioned as accompanying diphtheria, with the exception of the membrane. For instance, scarlet fever, quinsy sore throat, ulcerated sore throat, and common inflammatory sore throat from cold, may all be accompanied by soreness, difficulty of swallowing, pain in the throat and fever, while the ulcers in ulcerated sore throat may be easily mistaken for the membrane peculiar to diphtheria. On the contrary, diphtheria is sometimes, though rarely, unaccompanied by difficulty of swallowing. The most judicious way when there is a sudden attack of sore throat which is at all severe, is to consult a physician as speedily as possible, particularly if diphtheria is at all prevalent, as it is a disease which attacks both old and young ; young people being most liable to it. The number of cases of genuine diphtheria in proportion to the number of cases of other kinds of sore throat is extremely small; but when it does exist, a fatal termination can, in the majority of cases, be averted, if immediate treatment be entered upon. It may be stated simply as a matter of interest to the reader, that diphtheria may prove fatal by the membrane extending into the windpipe or larynx, and impeding respiration, or by extending into the nose and throat, or by the exhaustion, and severe character of the fever which generally accompanies the disease

TREATMENT.—As the above description has been given principally in order to assist in the recognition of the disease, and as the management of the disease should be entrusted to none but a physician, but little need be said in regard to the treatment. When from an examination of the throat the disease appears to exist, *Mercurius Solubilis* and *Belladonna* may, in a great majority of the cases, be given with advantage until medical aid can be obtained.

Dose, etc.—The two medicines may be given in alternation two hours apart. The dose of Mercurius Solubilis to an adult being five grains, to a child over two and under fifteen years of age, three or four grains The Belladonna is to be prepared by mixing 6 drops with half a tumbler of water of which the dose is a teaspoonful; for children from two to fifteen years of age, four drops may be added to half a glass of water. The diet should in all cases of diphtheria be as nourishing as possible, wine, wine-whey, beef tea, nourishing broths, &c., are necessary.

Dysentery.

Symptoms.—This disease may be recognized by the circumstances that *it is accompanied by straining and bearing down, with burning or soreness in the back passage; there is frequent inclination to go to stool, often unaccompanied by a passage or but a slight one, though somtimes the discharge is copious. The character of the stool varies, its most constant characteristic being that it contains more or less blood; the stools generally consist of a pure, jelly-like mucus, or mucus mixed with blood, or pure blood,* or they may be green, black or putrid.

There are also pain and tenderness on pressure, in the circumference of the bowels, and generally violent cutting or crampy pains. If the attack be severe or prolonged it is accompanied by more or less fever.

Causes.—It is most frequently caused by a change of temperature, a chill, moisture, &c., and is therefore most prevalent in the months of August and September when the days are warm and the nights cool. Other causes are such as may produce any disorder of the digestive organs, as unripe or stale fruit, &c.

TREATMENT.—If there be fever, commence the treatment with a dose of *Aconite*, prepared by adding five drops to half a tumbler of water, a teaspoonfull to be given at a dose. Then,

1. If the stools consist of mucus or mucus mixed with blood, accompanied by burning, soreness and straining at the anus; green, frothy, or sour smelling stools, fleshy, jelly-like stools, cutting pains in the bowels, chilliness and shivering, cold perspiration, soreness of the bowels, white coated tongue, give *Merc. Sol.*

DOSE.—Four or five grains every hour or two.

2. If there are very severe crampy or colicky pains in the bowels, and particularly if there are crampy or aching pains in the limbs, great relief may be obtained by giving *Coloc.* in alternation with the ***Merc. Sol.***, or with whatever remedy is most indicated. This remedy may also be administered when, with or without these symptoms, the evacuations are mucous, scanty, or slimy, or streaked with blood, or are watery, greenish, or yellow.

3. *When there is much discharge of blood, pure or mixed, Merc. Corr.* should be administered. This is the most valuable remedy we possess in the treatment of dysentery. It is particularly of value in autumnal dysentery, or when it proceeds from a chill.

The characteristic indications for its use, are frequent small passages of bloody mucus, or of chopped up looking greenish masses mixed with blood, fœtid or brownish mucus; constant and painful bearing down and inclination to go to stool without an evacuation, or with the evacuation of a little mucus; severe, cutting and griping pains, before, during, and after the motions; increased desire to go to stool after each evacuation; great thirst; sometimes oppression of the stomach and vomiting; the straining and evacuations are sometimes accompanied by protrusion of a portion of the intestines.

Dose.—Five grains for an adult, to be taken at a

dose, each dose to be dissolved in half a table-spoonful of water: to a child from five to ten years old, half that quantity may be given. A dose to be taken after each evacuation.

4. When the discharges *are dark brown, bilious looking*, copious, having a *fermented* look, with or without blood, accompanied by great and painful bearing down, burning, and great soreness and tenderness in the anus, cutting pains in the bowels, severe pain in its circumference, give *Aloes*.

DOSE.—Three drops to be added to half a tumbler of water. A teaspoonful to be given after each movement of the bowels.

5. When the attack is accompanied by high fever, hot, dry skin, thirst, bilious vomiting, with bearing down, or when there are rheumatic pains in the head or back of neck and shoulders, give *Aconite*. This remedy may be used with advantage *in conjunction* with other remedies, in all cases of dysentery accompanied by fever, and is valuable when the attack can be traced to a chill.

When there are bloody discharges, with bearing down and straining behind, and none of the remedies mentioned above give relief, *Ipecac* may be given in alternation with *Merc. Corr.*, or with *Merc. Sol.*, six drops being mixed with half a tumbler of water, of which the dose is a teaspoonful.

Diet, &c.—Keep the bowels and back wrapped warmly in flannel. *Give no solid food*; give nourishment enough simply to support the strength, which may be done by light preparations of barley water, gruel, sago, rice, arrow root, &c., or if the exhaustion be great, chicken broth or beef tea. This diet should be observed for some time after convalescence.

Earache.

Children as well as adults are subject to earache, proceeding in most cases from a cold or from "gatherings" or small abcesses in the ear. If the ear be examined by letting the patient sit with the head in such a position that the sunlight will fall directly upon it, the ear being pulled up at the top by the thumb and forefinger, so as to open it as much as possible, it will frequently be possible to ascertain whether or not there is a gathering, which is recognized by redness, swelling, or the presence of a small tumor in some part of the canal of the ear, or by the presence of water or matter. If there be nothing of this nature seen, give *Merc. Sol.* and *Belladonna*, according to the general directions for the administration of remedies on pages IX and X, and soak thoroughly a small piece of cotton in *Hamamelis*, which should first be warmed, and push it carefully into the ear; this should be changed every half hour or every hour, until the pain is relieved.

If the presence of a gathering be detected, *Merc. Sol.* and *Bell.* should be given as directed in the Introduction, and the Hamamelis employed in the same manner, and cloths, wrung out of hot water, kept applied over the ear. If there should be much matter however, cotton should not be introduced, as the discharge should have a free egress, but if there should be much pain the cloths may be applied. Generally, however, after the ear has commenced discharging, the pain ceases.

Epileptic Fits.

An attack of epilepsy generally comes on suddenly, though it may be preceded by various symptoms. In an attack of ordinary severity, the patient falls down suddenly, there are strong convulsive movements, spasmodic closure of the jaws, spasmodic twitching of the muscles of the face; the hands are clenched, there is difficult, choking respiration, foaming at the mouth, and the face becomes turgid or blue, while the veins of the forehead and neck are swollen and distended. The spasmodic state becomes at length gradually less, gives way, and is followed by deep sleep.

Diagnosis.—It is important that an epileptic fit should not be mistaken for an attack of apoplexy, as entirely different treatment is required for the two. The marks of distinction will be found on page 15.

TREATMENT.—All that need be done during the attack, is to prevent the patient injuring himself. Place the patient on the back, *the head being somewhat elevated*, loosen all articles of clothing about the neck, and if the fit be severe, place if possible a small bit of wood or a small roll of cotton or muslin between the teeth, to prevent the tongue from being bitten. Cold water may also be sprinkled on the face and chest.

Inflammation of the Eyes.

These directions for the eye refer not to severe or chronic affections of this organ, but to inflammation and pain produced by cold, wind, etc., etc.—*catarrhal* inflammation of the eyes. They are red, painful, sensitive to the light, discharge water profusely, and there may be a discharge of matter.

TREATMENT.—Give *Stibium* and *Belladonna* in alternation, two hours apart. Cold or warm water, as may be most agreeable to the patient, may be kept applied part of the time by means of linen cloths, to the eyes, or the eyes may be bathed occasionally. A physician should be consulted, if the trouble should be severe, as local applications may be required.

Should there be much pain in and above the eyes, *Arsenicum* and *Stibium* may be given.

DOSES, ETC.—See page VIII.

Fainting.

Treatment.—Place patient on the back, the head *low*; give plenty of fresh air by opening a window; do not crowd around her; sprinkle the face with a little cold water; loosen the dress about the chest; apply salts or hartshorn to the nostrils, and as soon as she can swallow, give a little brandy or wine.

Where fainting occurs, however, after or during severe bleeding, or flooding, do not try to revive the patient, unless the swoon lasts some time.

Headaches

Are so variable in their character, and are due to such a variety of causes, that only a few directions for the most common forms will be given.

Like all other affections, headache should be treated, as far as possible, with reference to its cause. The most common varieties are *rheumatic*, situated in the muscular covering of the head—a species of rheumatism of the scalp, always produced by cold; *neuralgic*, produced in most cases by cold; *congestive*, produced by disordered circulation of the vessels of the brain; and *dyspeptic* or *sympathetic*, probably the most common form, dependent upon some disorder of the digestive system, dyspepsia, constipation, disorder of the liver, derangements of the monthly sickness, &c., &c.

The rheumatic may be recognized by the pain extending over the head, and by being accompanied often by pain in the neck, face, shoulders, &c.

The neuralgic, by its occurring often, at certain times or periods, by generally affecting one side of the face or head, or the eyes, nose, and jaws.

The sympathetic may be surmised from the existence of any of the disorders above referred to.

TREATMENT.—The principal remedies for headaches are:

Aconite and *Bryonia*, in headaches from cold or disorders of the liver.

Bell., in nervous, neuralgic, sympathetic, or congestive headaches, and headaches from disorders of the monthly sickness.

Nux. Vom. in nervous headaches, headaches from disorders of the liver or digestive system, *sick headaches*.

Ignatia, in nervous headaches.

Arsenicum, in headaches from cold, or disorders of the stomach.

Aconite and *Bryonia* may be given, particularly in headaches proceeding from exposure to cold, accompanied by fulness of head, fever, red face, chilliness; pain extending down the neck; pain in the limbs or shoulders; *soreness* of the head and tenderness on pressure; fullness of the head and forehead; pressure and weight in the forehead; soreness of the eyes; numbness and stupefaction of the head, as if it were compressed on all sides; shooting pains in head; great nervousness and irritability; pain increased by the slightest movement.

The characteristic symptoms of headache to which *Belladonna* is suited, are pain in the forehead and aching in the eyes; redness of the eyes and flow of tears; pain increased by light or noise; feeling as if the skull would be pressed open; heaviness of the head; headache in the forehead, as if the brain would be pressed out; headache, accompanied by shooting pains; stitches and lacerating pains in the head; violent, tearing, bursting, cutting pains; pains on top of the head; lacerating pains over the eyes; headache, confined entirely to or worse on one side of the head; great restlessness; patient almost unconscious or almost distracted from the pain; violent throbbing; redness of face; giddiness; fever; beating pain; throbbing in temples; pain on the right side of the back and spine. *Aconite* and *Bell.* may often be given with benefit, in alternation, particularly if febrile or rheumatic symptoms are present.

DOSE.—Five drops of *Bell.* to half a tumbler of water. A teaspoonful from every half hour to two hours.

Nux. Vomica should be employed in headache proceeding from disorders of the stomach or liver; suppressed bleeding from piles; too much coffee; from over-eating, mental labor, or anxiety; in nervous headaches, and headaches in hysterical subjects; in bilious headaches; in headaches accompanied by ***great irritability;*** by dizziness, confusion of ideas, stupefaction; faintness, with congestion of the head and redness of the face, particularly if produced by any of the causes mentioned above; throbbing, beating headache; scalp tender, and sore to the touch; head feels bruised; headache on top of the head; headache confined to one side of the head—shooting, piercing, confined perhaps to one spot; feeling as if the brain were cleft; lacerating pain in the forehead; head heavy and sore, feeling as if a nail were driven into the head; pale face, weakness, trembling, sudden starting.

DOSE.—Five drops to be mixed with half a tumbler of water; a teaspoonful to be given from every half hour to every two hours.

From the above symptoms, it may be seen that the headaches for which *Nux.* is recommended are similar in many respects to the varieties in which *Bell.* is directed, and it may seem difficult in some cases to determine which of the two remedies to employ. They have, indeed, many points in common; both are suited to congestive headaches; both to lacerating, throbbing pains, and pains in the forehead; and both to headaches, accompanied by redness in the face. The following marks of distinction will however prove a sufficient guide in making the selection:

Belladonna is suited particularly to headaches of individuals of a full habit; to *females*; to individuals with light hair, blue eyes, delicate skin, and is especially of use when the headache is due to a suppression or non-appearance of the monthly illness.

Nux Vomica more particularly to bilious or nervous temperaments; to males; to persons with pale or red face; to persons subject to piles; to headaches from disorders of the liver, stomach, or from constipation or mental disorders, anxiety, &c. A careful comparison of the difference of the symptoms and of their circumstances will generally lead to a correct choice. *Bell.* is however *more* suited to congestive headaches, or where there is a great rush of blood to the head or face. There are cases in which *both* may be used with the greatest advantage: for example, which seem to combine the symptoms of the two remedies, as suppressed bleeding from piles, or dyspeptic symptoms in very plethoric individuals.

Ignatia is invaluable in *purely nervous headaches*, and to headaches occurring in hysterical or very sensitive people, particularly females; to headaches accompanied by palpitation of the heart, restlessness, inclination to shed tears, depression of spirits; together with the above characteristics, the symptoms of headache proper, for which it is suited, are painful pressure, either in the forehead or back of the head, or it may exist all over the head; the pain changes about to different parts; pain in the eyes; boring, sticking pain in the forehead, over the root of the nose; feeling as if a sharp body were pressed into the brain; great irritability; burning and sensitiveness of the eyes, dimness of sight, or increased by noise.

Dose—Four drops in half a tumbler of water; a tea-spoonful of which may be given from half an hour to two hours apart.

When there is dull, heavy, stupefying pain; buzzing, throbbing, tightness; headache worse after eating, accompanied by nausea, retching or dizziness; headache confined to one side of the head; burning in the scalp; *pain and aching in the eyes and over the root of the nose; flow of tears and burning in the eyes, with redness of the eyes and catarrh;* dimness of sight; eyes sensitive to the light; severe pain in the forehead; aching in the eyeballs; *Arsenicum* should be used. This remedy is of particular value if the latter symptoms are the result of cold; also in rheumatic headaches; in headaches from disordered digestion from eating rich food. In catarrhal headaches it may be given in alternation with *Bell.*; in headaches characterized by the symptoms and caused by disorders of the stomach, it may be given in alternation with ***Nux. Vomica.*** Arsenicum and Nux. Vomica may be also given in alternation in "sick headache,".with great benefit.

DOSE, ADMINISTRATION, ETC.—Each of the above medicines is to be prepared by mixing five drops with half a glass of water. If two remedies are given, they may be taken in alternation, from one to two hours apart, in teaspoonful doses.

Intoxication—Drunkenness.

A fit of intoxication may be of such a character as to require speedy medical interference. Drunken fits have sometimes been mistaken for the more respectable diseases of apoplexy, epilepsy, and poisoning by opium, and have been treated accordingly, to the great detriment of the patient. When a person is "dead drunk," the trouble might be mistaken for poisoning by opium, as the two conditions often resemble each other closely, and are both accompanied by stupor. Intoxication may be generally recognized by the odor of the breath, the patient's habits, the circumstances in which he is found, &c.

TREATMENT.—A liberal supply of fresh air should be obtained by opening the doors and windows. If there be obstinate insensibility and stupor, the patient should be laid on his back with the head to one side to favor vomiting, which should be excited by tickling the back part of the throat with a feather or with the finger; should that not produce vomiting, an emetic should be given; an emetic almost always at hand is common mustard, of which two or three teaspoonfuls may be given, mixed with half a tumbler of warm water; should this not act, fifteen grains of the *Sulphate of Zinc* dissolved in water, may be given. The action of the emetics may be promoted by dashing cold water on the head and face.

A handkerchief moistened with hartshorn may also be held before the nose, and fifteen to twenty drops mixed with water, may be given internally. When the stupor and prostration have yielded, ***Nux Vomica*** may be given.

DOSE.—Five drops may be mixed with half a tumbler of water, and a tea-spoonful given from every half hour to every two hours.

Threatened Miscarriage.

CAUSES.—Over exertion, fatigue, mental emotions, the habit of miscarrying, debility, etc.

SYMPTOMS.—Sometimes a miscarriage will take

place with scarcely any symptoms. Generally however it is preceded or accompanied by pains in the back, loins or in the bowels, sometimes cutting or colicky, and sometimes bearing down. Greater or less discharge of mucus or blood may also be present.

TREATMENT.—Let the patient keep her bed; the diet should be light; cold drinks, lemonade, &c., may be taken, and the *greatest possible quiet observed*, until the symptoms have passed off.

Internally *Coloc.* and *Cham.* may be taken in alternation from one to two hours apart. These remedies are of use before the symptoms are severe, and will frequently check their development. If the symptoms are severe or if there be a discharge of mucus or blood, medical assistance should be sent for. These remedies however may be continued until medical advice can be obtained. Patients should not, unless they are obliged to, attempt to treat a case of this kind, without assistance. The above directions, &c., are given as they may prevent a *threatened* miscarriage, or serve for the management of one when it is inevitable, until the arrival of a physician.

DOSES.—Five drops of each of the medicines above mentioned to be mixed with half a glass of water of which a teaspoonful is to be taken at a dose.

Non-appearance or delay of the Monthly Sickness May be owing to various conditions. It may be the result of cold, of pregnancy, of constitutional debility, of plethora ; these being the most frequent causes. When it is due to either of the two last mentioned causes, generally a regular course of treatment is necessary, to restore the regularity of the monthly flow, and often, medical assistance, to bring it on at all. When either of these two conditions exist, if there be *any* irregularity in this function, it will be likely to occur repeatedly, or the monthly sickness may be absent for a long time. The treatment must therefore be principally constitutional. When however its non-appearance is owing to having taken cold or when it has *previously* been regular and no cause can be assigned for its non-appearance, it may often be brought on by taking, if it be accompanied by fullness of the head, redness of the face, headache, *Belladonna* and *Pulsatilla*, in alternation two hours apart.

If these symptoms of the head are absent, give *Puls.* and *Nux.*, two hours apart.

Doses.—Each of these medicines is to be prepared by mixing 5 drops in half a tumbler of water, of which the dose is a teaspoonfull. In addition to these remedies the hot foot bath, hip bath, warm drinks, and the other measures directed in the article following on suppression of the monthly sickness, may be resorted to for several nights in succession. The patient should be warmly dressed, and cold should be avoided as much as possible.

Suppression of the Monthly Sickness.

If the monthly flow has been stopped suddenly from cold or other causes, after it has commenced, take *Aconite* and *Pulsatilla* in alternation an hour and a half apart until it returns. A foot bath of hot water should also be taken at bed time to which should be added a tablespoonful of mustard. A warm hip bath may also be taken with advantage, and warm drinks as tea or gruel, be taken internally. The patient should go to bed, and warmth promoted in every way.

Should there be much fullness, throbbing or pain in the head, *Aconite*, *Pulsatilla* and *Belladonna* may be taken in alternation an hour apart.

DOSE, etc.—Each of these medicines is to be prepared by mixing 6 drops with half a tumbler of water, and given in teaspoonful doses.

Neuralgia of the Face and Head

Is so common, that it does not need a very minute description. It consists of severe pains of the nerves of the head or face, or both; sometimes the pain extends into the jaw, sometimes into the eye and forehead, sometimes the whole of one side of the head is affected, the pain extending even to the spine or shoulder, the pain is sharp, shooting, aching, or burning, and in many cases returns at regular periods or intervals. If the eye is affected there is a profuse flow of tears.

CAUSES.—The most common is cold, decayed teeth and disorders of the monthly sickness.

TREATMENT.—In neuralgia proceeding from cold, accompanied by burning and pain in or about the eye or in the temples, or at the root of the nose, with flow of tears, catarrh, or pain in the jaw, *Ars.* should be given.

DOSE.—For an adult, 5 drops to be mixed with half a tumbler of water, of which a teaspoonfull is to be taken at a dose. The dose for other ages in proportion to the age. See pages IX–X.

In neuralgia with pain confined to one side of the head or face, attended with tearing, darting pains in the jaws or teeth, pains in the eyes, temples or forehead, with redness of the face, violent headache, stiffness of the neck, *Bell.* is the remedy.

DOSE.—Same as *Ars.* above.

When there are soreness of the head, soreness of the teeth, burning, shooting, swelling of the glands under the jaws or teeth, especially if they are decayed; pain worse after going to bed, chilliness, perspiration, *Merc. Sol.* should be taken in alternation with *Cham.*, half an hour to an hour apart.

DOSE.—For an adult, as much *Merc.* as will lie on an old-fashioned silver three-cent piece (about five grains). For dose for children, see page IX. *Cham.* should be prepared, ten or fifteen drops of *Cham.*, to be mixed with half a glass of water. Dose, a tea-spoonful.

Aconite should be resorted to in neuralgia from cold, with fever, rheumatic pains, alternate heat and chills, throbbing, burning, swelling of the face.

DOSE.—See page VIII.

It will frequently be necessary to give *two* of the above remedies, in alternation from one to two hours apart, or even oftener if the pain should be severe, until relief is obtained. For instance *Ars.* and *Bell.* *Bell* and *Merc. Sol.*; *Aconite* and *Merc. Sol.* may be given in alternation, according as the symptoms experienced by the patient correspond to the symptoms described above. Aconite may always be given with advantage alone, or in conjunction with another remedy, when there is fever.

Another means of relief of great value in neuralgia of the face, and toothache, is a mustard poultice applied to the face, and made by mixing thoroughly one teaspoonful of English mustard with six of Indian meal, wet with hot water, and gradually adding to this and mixing six teaspoonfuls of flour. It should be applied hot between two pieces of thin muslin and may be allowed to remain on any length of time as it will not blister nor irritate the skin.

Rheumatism.

This disease may require such a variety of remedies and often such diligent treatment, that only a few remedies will be given, intended for the treatment of the affection as soon as it makes its appearance and before a severe attack is developed; but not for cases of rheumatism of long standing.

TREATMENT.—For rheumatic pains arising from cold, check of perspiration, etc., characterized by aching pains all over, chilliness, lameness, and for rheumatic pains generally, *without perspiration*, *Aconite* and *Merc. Sol.* should be given two hours apart.

DOSES.—Six drops of the *Aconite* to be mixed with half a glass of water, of which the dose is a tea-spoonful. The dose of the *Merc. Sol.* is as much as will lie heaped up on a silver three-cent piece.

When the symptoms are of the same nature as described above, and are *accompanied by perspiration*, *Colchicum* and *Mercurius Solubilis*, are the remedies, an hour or two apart.

DOSES.—Same as *Aconite* and *Merc.* above.

When the joints are red and swollen, *Colchicum* should be taken every two hours. If accompanied by fever, *Aconite* should be taken in alternation with it, two hours apart.

DOSES, ETC —See Introduction, page VII.

If the pains are relieved by moving about or by motion, *Rhus.* should be taken.

DOSE, ETC.—See page VIII.

For rheumatic pains in the shoulder—sharp or sore pains, pains in the chest, particularly in taking a long breath, Colchicum and Rhus should be taken two hours apart.

DOSES, ETC.—See page. VIII.

Sea Sickness.

The remedies and expedients recommended in this complaint are innumerable.

A dose of *Nux. Vom.*, may be taken with advantage on an empty stomach 12 hours and 6 hours before sailing; as soon as nausea sets in, *Ars.* and *Nux* may be taken in alternation from one to three hours apart.

When the sickness becomes excessive, is attended with violent retching, prostration, and burning in the throat, *Ars.* may be given in alternation with *Nux.*

DOSES, ETC.—See page VIII.

When the above remedies are insufficient, 10 or 12 drops of Chloroform may be given in water, two or three times a day if necessary. Capsules each containing three or four drops of chloroform are kept by druggists, and are a very convenient way of taking this remedy.

Keep on the back the first twenty-four or forty-eight hours of the voyage, and after that keep on deck as much as possible. Avoid all alcoholic stimulants generally, except iced champagne. Great care should be taken to avoid rich food. A bowl of oat-meal gruel may be always taken with advantage before rising.

PART II.

THE TREATMENT OF CASES OF POISONING.

Accidental cases of poisoning are most liable to occur from ACONITE, ARSENIC, CORROSIVE SUBLIMATE, OPIUM and TARTAR EMETIC, as these poisons are often kept in the house for various purposes.

Poisoning by Aconite.

The tincture and other preparations of this plant are frequently administered by physicians for various diseases. It is a poison producing great prostration and weakness, and loss of power, both of the nervous and muscular systems; sometimes producing paralysis of the organs of respiration, and a deadening of all the faculties.

TREATMENT.—I. Evacuate the stomach by an emetic. 30 grains of the Sulphate of Zinc may be given for this purpose, dissolved in warm water. After vomiting has been produced, give stimulants —brandy or ammonia, (hartshorn,) 15 to 20 drops of the latter, mixed with water, and repeated from time to time.

If there are spasms, the warm bath should be resorted to.

Arsenic.

The symptoms of poisoning by Arsenic vary according to the amount taken. The most prominent are nausea, vomiting, retching, cold extremities, trembling, weakness, anxiety, chills, burning in the throat and mouth, violent or unquenchable thirst, diarrhœa, purging, colicky, crampy pains, sometimes fainting, and collapse, (these two symptoms rare,) and sometimes spasms.

These symptoms vary in the degree of their intensity, often being less strongly marked, and sometimes much more violent. In severe cases, every organ and function of the body may be affected.

TREATMENT.—The first step to be taken in domestic practice is to free the stomach from the poison by producing vomiting, (*if vomiting has not set in of itself.*) Do this by tickling the throat with the finger, or with a feather, if this do not prove sufficient, two or three spoonfuls of mustard may be given with half a tumbler of water; or 20 or 30 grains of the sulphate of zinc may be given dissolved in a little water. The emetic best suited however to poisoning by Arsenic, is a tea made by steeping a common small paper of tobacco, or if that be not at hand one or two cigars broken up, in a teacupfull of water; of this a teaspoonful may be given at a dose every five or ten minutes until vomiting commences, when it should be discontinued, as it is a remedy apt to produce great prostration.

Tartar Emetic should never be given in cases of poisoning by Arsenic.

After vomiting has taken place, one of the following remedies is to be given. They are arranged in the order of their value.

1. Let the patient swallow pulverized charcoal.
2. If that be not at hand give sweet oil plentifully.
3. Calcined magnesia mixed to the thickness of cream, in doses of two or three tablespoonfuls. After the violent symptoms have been subdued, beef tea, strengthening broths, wine and water may be given.

Corrosive Sublimate.

In poisoning by corrosive sublimate, give at once the *white* of several eggs. These are the best domestic antidote; the white of one egg is enough to antidote four grains of the poison; if the eggs are not at hand, give until they can be obtained flour mixed with water, or in place of that let the patient drink milk. After having given this antidote induce vomiting by draughts of lukewarm water, tickling the throat with a feather, &c. Should these not produce vomiting, give 20 or 30 grains of the sulphate of zinc in a little water.

Poisoning by Sulphuric Acid, Oil of Vitriol, Vitriol.

Give magnesia and water, the carbonate of soda, potash and water, or chalk and water. If these are not at hand, give oil, milk, flour and water, ashes and water or pure water. Flax seed or slippery elm tea, may also be given.

If external parts be burned, wash with soap and water.

Nitric Acid, (Aqua Fortis.)

Same antidotes as for sulphuric acid.

Hydrochloric Acid, Muriatic Acid.

Give magnesia and water, chalk and water, carbonate of soda or potash and water; whiting scraped from the wall in the absence of any of the above remedies, which are named in the order of their value. Next to these, oil, white of eggs, flour and water and milk, are valuable; these last named remedies should be given in *large quantities*, in case of poisoning by any of the acids.

Opium, Laudanum, Paregoric, Godfrey's Cordial, Morphine.

Opium, and the above preparations of it, are narcotic poisons, producing in over doses giddiness, heaviness, stupor, insensibility, slow, labored breathing, the face is generally pale and the patient lies quite still as if in a deep sleep.

TREATMENT.—Give an emetic of from 20 to 30

grains of the Sulphate of Zinc, in a little water. The dose must be proportioned to the amount of stupor or insensibility. For an adult, 30 grains should be given at once. For the doses for an infant, see pages 11–12. If this do not produce vomiting in 5 or 10 minutes, give strong black coffee, as strong as it can be made. This will often produce vomiting when all other means fail, though if this should fail, a second dose of sulphate of zinc may be given.

Should vomiting however *not* be brought on by either of these remedies, give a tablespoonful of saleratus or soda in water, and immediately after a tumbler full of vinegar and water as strong as it can be taken without scalding the throat; vomiting may be assisted after either of the above remedies, by tickling the back part of the throat with a feather or the finger. Do do not, however, give all these emetics at once. Commence with the one first directed, and if it do not act after a proper time has elapsed, give another, and so on.

After the emetic has been given, employ every possible means to rouse the patient; dash cold water, or cold and warm water in alternation upon the chest, neck and face; give stimulants internally, strong coffee with a little brandy in it, &c. After vomiting, give acid drinks, as vinegar and water, or lemon juice.

As long as the drowsiness continues the patient should not be suffered to give way to it, but should be walked up and down the room between two persons.

Sometimes after a large quantity of laudanum or its preparations has been taken, respiration appears to have ceased entirely, and the patient seems dead. When this condition exists or when the patient does not swallow, even when the substances administered are placed far back on the tongue :

1. Pour water, as cold as can be procured, from a height upon the spine.

2. If this produce no return of animation, *artificial respiration* must be resorted to. This is performed as follows :

1. Place the patient on the face upon a table; then turn the body on the side and a little beyond, then briskly on the face or breast again, and so from the side to the face alternately, once in about four or five seconds. The side on which the patient is turned should be varied occasionally.

2. Each time the body is placed on the face, make uniform but firm pressure *between and below the shoulder blades*, on *each side of the spine*, removing the pressure immediately before turning the body on the side.

3. The head should project over the head of the

table, and the fingers should be occasionally introduced into the back part of the throat to excite vomiting.

As soon as there are signs of returning animation, an emetic should be given as first directed, and the treatment then pursued as afterwards directed.

Tartar Emetic

Produces in over doses, cramps, spasms, convulsions, vomiting, purging, and colicky pains.

TREATMENT.—1. Give strong green tea, as strong as it can be made ; to an infant, a few teaspoonfuls will suffice.

2. Chalk or magnesia, mixed with water to about the consistence of cream, may then be given.

3. If there is great prostration, a little brandy or wine may be administered.

4. If there are severe cramps, to an adult, from thirty to fifty drops of laudanum may be given.

PART III.

OF ACCIDENTS.

The General Treatment of Accidents, Falls, Injuries, Collapse, &c.

Numerous accidents are liable to occur, in which certain immediate measures may be of great use and are sometimes indispensable to the welfare of the patient, and as they may occur at any time, a few directions as to their immediate management will be of use. Among these are injuries received from falls; from being run over or knocked down by a passing vehicle; injuries received from cars; from blows by heavy bodies; where part of the body is crushed; or a limb broken; wounds from fire-arms; from explosions, &c.

Severe accidents of this kind are generally followed by a condition of prostration or collapse, due to the sudden shock given to the nervous system. The symptoms of the shock vary from simple faintness to complete insensibility; the patient, when the shock is severe, lying cold and breathless, with a feeble pulse, and wholly or partially unconscious.

Sometimes an *unimportant* and *slight* injury will

produce great collapse. Soldiers in action have fallen down from being simply grazed by a bullet, and others from merely thinking themselves shot. When the prostration is principally the effect of nervous fear, a little brandy or wine, and a few encouraging words will be sufficient to restore the patient.

When it is owing to severe injury, other methods must be resorted to :

1. Place the patient in a comfortable position, with the head low, unless it be the seat of the injury, and the wounded part so that it will be favorably situated and so as to be as little painful as possible. Then, if the prostration be great and there is perfect insensibility and there are no signs of *reaction*, stimulants should be resorted to. Frictions should be employed over the surface of the body ; injections containing brandy, or prepared by beating up the spirits of turpentine with the yolk of an egg and mixing it with water, may be administered ; hot bricks or bottles of hot water should be applied under the arm pits, and to the feet ; the body should be wrapped up warmly, and ammonia (hartshorn) may be applied to the nostrils. Care must be taken however not to employ this last remedy too freely, as injury is often done by it.

As soon as the patient can swallow, give a little wine and water or a little tea.

Care must be taken however not to *overstimulate* the patient, as the danger of too great reaction or return of the vital powers is often more to be feared than collapse.

In injuries to the *head* particularly, care should be taken not to stimulate too much, as these injuries are very liable to be followed by inflammatory conditions of the brain.

If there be not complete insensibility, but only great prostration, give stimulants sufficient simply to keep up the patient.

Finally, in all injuries, place the patient and the injured part in as comfortable a position as possible; if an arm be broken lay it straight by the patient's side, or support it on a pillow; if a leg, place the patient on the back with the leg extended; if an arm or **leg** be thought to be badly injured, do not attempt to *draw* off the clothing, but cut it carefully away.

The Treatment of Particular Accidents.

Bites and Stings of Insects.

These little things are not only painful, but sometimes even dangerous. In stings of bees or wasps, or even mosquitoes, when very painful, extract the sting if left in the wound. This may often be done by applying a watch key over it and pressing firmly upon it. The best local application is tobacco moistened in a little water. Brandy, sweet oil, turpentine, cologne water, &c., will be found beneficial.

Dr. Hill of Cleveland, recommends as the result of repeated trials. the application of a raw onion to the sting. The onion to be cut in two and the surface to be kept applied, changing it every ten or fifteen minutes until the pain and swelling disappear. He considers it certain to procure relief.

Bites of Mad Dogs.—Hydrophobia.

It is of the utmost importance to be able to determine at an *early period* when a dog is affected with the disease known as Hydrophobia, or more properly *rabies* (madness), but sometimes, to one unacquainted with the symptoms of the disease, it is not only very difficult, but impossible.

I subjoin therefore, a description of the symptoms as they commonly appear, the main points of which are derived principally from "Youatt on the Dog."

In the early stages, there are sullenness, fidgitiness and continual change of posture, and an extreme degree of restlessness. Frequently he is almost invariably wandering about, shifting from corner to corner, or continually rising up or lying down; changing his posture in every possible way; disposing of his bed with his paws, shaking it up with his mouth, &c. He begins to gaze strangely about him ; his countenance is clouded and suspicious. If at liberty he will seem to imagine that something is lost, and will search eagerly round the room, particularly in every corner of it, with strange violence and indecision.

The attachment of the dog to his master may be in the earliest stages very much increased, and he is employed, almost without ceasing, in licking the hands or whatever part he can get at. Sometimes the appetite is altered or depraved, the dog seeming disgusted with his food, and at others seizing it with his usual avidity, and often chewing it a little and dropping it as if unable to swallow it. This is almost a certain sign of madness. The dog works at his mouth with his paws, as if there were a bone there which he endeavors to dislodge. Sometimes he flies at inanimate objects and endeavors to tear them to pieces, biting at nails, the walls, &c.

The voice is changed, being either hoarse, or pitched on a higher key than is natural. The idea that there is profuse and constant foaming at the mouth is erroneous, the saliva being secreted profusely for a period of only about twelve hours. Sometimes, when the attack is fully developed, the dog shows no inclination to bite, seeming as if sick and tired, and suffering persons to handle him gently; in other cases the ferocity of the animal knows no bounds; dogs have been known to pick up hot coals of fire and chew them, and to hold red hot pokers in the mouth. If a dog in this state of madness makes his escape, he rushes all over, biting whatever animal or man comes in his way.

There is also *excessive thirst*, the dog wanting to drink constantly and freely. In one or two cases this has been almost the only symptom. In most cases the dog swallows easily, but in others, though devoured by thirst, he is unable to swallow a drop, owing to the swelling and paralysis of the muscles of the throat. When the muscles of the mouth and throat are thus affected, the mouth is partly open and the tongue partly protruded.

It is the *saliva* of the mad dog which is poisonous, and which gets into the wound made by the bite. It is not a little dangerous, therefore, to be licked by a mad dog, since if the saliva come in contact with any wound, sore, scratch or abrasion, or even with a pimple, the poison may be admitted into the system.

This disease is not limited to the dog; any animal may be affected with it, though when it exists in other animals, it generally comes from infection from the dog.

SEASON, CAUSES, ETC.—Rabies commonly occurs in the warm months of the year, though it may occur even in winter. It is caused, when not owing to the bite of mad animals, most frequently by confinement, improper food, &c.

How soon, after the bite is received, *does the disease show itself in the system?* is an important question. Generally in from three to five months. There is one instance recorded, where the system became affected in fourteen days after; another, not until twelve, and another *thirty* years after. The last two cases are extremely doubtful. If the disease does not show itself by the end of six months, there is not much danger of its ever making its appearance.

TREATMENT.—The bite should be cauterized as soon as possible by the solid Nitrate of Silver (Lunar Caustic). A piece, the shape of a pencil or pointed, should be pressed firmly into the bite and twisted around so that every part may be reached, and until it seems thoroughly *burned out*. The nitrate of siver is the best application; next in value come pure nitric acid, caustic potash, and last, red hot iron. After the wound has been thus treated, it should be *cut out*. This can be done properly only by a medical man. Sucking the wound, and putting a ligature above it, are of little use; the former is dangerous, as there might be some fissure about the lips by which the poison might enter.

Bite of the Rattlesnake.

The most certain remedy for the bite of the rattlesnake is some one of the alcoholic preparations:—whisky [this is the best], rum, gin, brandy, etc. It should be taken at short intervals, and in considerable quantities, until intoxication is produced. Alcoholic preparations, taken in sufficient quantities, may be regarded almost as a certain antidote to the bite of the rattlesnake.

The wound should be also instantly cauterized by the nitrate of silver, as directed in the preceding article on the bite of the mad dog.

I am not aware that the alcoholic preparations have been employed in the treatment of the bite of other snakes than the rattlesnake, but should consider them worthy of a trial.

The local application of strong spirits of hartshorn, together with its internal administration, has averted a fatal termination after the bite of some snakes, particularly the Cobra de Capello. It should be given internally in doses of from 10 to 20 drops in water, every five or ten minutes, until several doses have been given. When used externally, it should be applied very freely.

Bleeding—Hæmorrhage.

1. From wounds.—In cases of bleeding, no matter how profuse, do not be alarmed nor lose presence of mind, but remember that the most profuse bleed-

ing can be subdued to a great extent by resorting to the proper means, at least until medical assistance can be obtained, and that bleeding from an accidental wound rarely proves fatal, though no accident produces more alarm in the minds of lookers on.

TREATMENT, DIRECTIONS, &c.—Do not cover up the wound with handkerchiefs, towels, bandages, &c. First ascertain the source of the bleeding. Hæmorrhage or bleeding from a wound proceeds from one of two sources: First, from an artery, recognizable by the blood flowing in jets or by jerks, and by being of a bright red color. Second, from a vein, recognizable by the blood *oozing* or *welling* out, and being of a dark color.

Examine the wound carefully, and remove all dirt, clots, &c. 1. Then, if the bleeding be slight or proceed from a slight wound, there being but a simple oozing of blood, it may often be checked by the application of cloths wet with cold water, by pounded ice in linen cloths, or by raising the part in an elevated position; or cobwebs, the down from a hat, or powdered alum, or cotton may be applied. These methods will frequently arrest the bleeding when it proceeds from a bleeding surface, large or small in extent, but not accompanied with wounds of any large blood vessels.

2. When large blood vessels are cut open and the

flow of blood is profuse, there is more danger, and other measures must be resorted to:

1. Apply one or more fingers upon the point whence the blood flows, not *near* it, but if possible directly *upon* the mouth of the bleeding vessel, at the point where the blood can be seen or felt to gush out. If it can be seen, and it be possible, pinch the end of the bleeding vessel between the thumb and finger; if this cannot be done, or if the wound be over a bone, as on the head or forehead or on the arm, make firm pressure with one or two fingers upon the ends of the bleeding vessel or upon the bleeding point, pressing it against the bone. The bleeding may generally be restrained in this manner until medical assistance arrives.

Supposing, however, a large vessel to have been wounded and the flow of blood to be profuse, additional security will be found in the application of what is known as the *tourniquet*. The most common form of the instrument consists of a band made to encircle the whole limb, and having a pad placed under it to press upon the bleeding vessel. One may easily be made by tying a knot firmly in the middle of a cravat, or pocket handkerchief folded like a cravat; bind this around the limb a little above the wound, so that the knot will be directly over the blood vessel to be compressed; under the knot a compress about an inch square, of linen or cotton cloth, and made as hard as possible, may be placed. The two ends of the handkerchief are then to be tied together upon the limb, and a stick being inserted into the knot, it may be twisted so that the whole limb may be firmly compressed.

This will be of great use also when the fingers become cramped or unsteady. Do not, however, twist the stick so tightly as to prevent the circulation entirely; try to concentrate the pressure on the bleeding vessel.

The pressure should be made upon the blood vessel above the wound. The situation of the blood vessel can often be recognized by finding a pulsating point above the wound. In wounds of the arm pressure should be made on the inside of the arm against the bone; in wounds of the thigh, just inside the thigh at its commencement, on about the center.

The main artery of every limb runs downward along the inside of the limb.

3. If the bleeding seem to proceed from rather a large surface or from several small vessels, or there be a deep wound and so extensive that it cannot be checked by the means described in verse 1, pressure by pads or compresses must be resorted to.

This is to be done in the following manner: First remove all dirt, clots, or foreign bodies. Then place the finger on the bleeding point, and removing it, apply a small piece of lint, just large enough to cover it. Over this, place another little larger, and so on, layer after layer, firmly upon each other, each a little larger than the other, till the whole wound has been filled up a little higher than the surrounding skin. The compress will thus have the shape of a pyramid, of which the point will rest upon the wound, and the base will be a little above the level of the wound. Over this may be drawn a cravat, handkerchief, or bandage, so as to keep it firmly in its place and make some degree of pressure upon it, or strips of plaster may be drawn over it in different directions.

If the compress remain tolerably dry, it is a sign that the bleeding is checked. If on the contrary, the blood oozes through in considerable quantities, the compress must be undone, and reapplied more carefully and firmly.

If this do not prove effectual, use pressure with the fingers, and apply the tourniquet until assistance is obtained.

In bleeding from wounds caused by fire arms, or from *small* and *deep* wounds, it is impossible generally to apply compresses as described. In these cases the tourniquet should be employed, and the fingers applied firmly upon the upper and lower edge of bleeding orifice.

Bleeding from Leech Bites.

The bleeding from leech bites is sometimes very profuse, and, unless proper measures are taken, difficult to arrest. The following measures will be found efficacious.

Roll a small piece of the downy portion of lint into a hard ball a little smaller than a pea, wipe the bleeding orifice dry, and press the ball upon it. Then draw firmly over it a piece of adhesive plaster, so that it will extend an inch or two beyond it in each direction. A still more effectual method is, after bringing the edges of the little wound in contact, to unite them by means of two or three stitches with a fine needle and thread. Ice, locally applied, is very useful. Should this, however, not stop the bleeding, or if the bite be where the pressure or plaster cannot be applied, as on the eyelid, take the downy portion of lint, make a small hard ball almost the size of a pin's head, or large enough to fit closely into the orifice, wet this in a strong solution of alum, and, with the assistance of a pin or knitting-needle, press it into the orifice, first having wiped it quite dry.

Bleeding from leech bites may be restrained also by wiping the orifice dry, and then pinching together for ten or fifteen minutes the integument on each side of it, thus closing it completely.

Bruises. Contusions.

Keep the bruised part constantly wet by means of a linen rag, with a mixture of three or four teaspoonfuls of tincture of Arnica to a tumbler of water.

Burns and Scalds.

If the burn produce simply redness of the skin without the formation of blisters, and is slight in extent, cold water or ice may be kept constantly applied until the pain is relieved; or a cold poultice of grated potatoe or turnip may be applied till the pain abates. These applications must however be changed often enough to keep up the sensation of cold. After the pain abates the part may be warmly covered with soft cotton wool.

2. Soap lather made from a common shaving box may be applied coat after coat and allowed to dry on. Additional protection will be found in covering this with cotton wool, (cotton batting.)

3. An invaluable remedy in burns, not attended with the formation of blisters, even if they be quite extensive, is the liquid collodion. Several coats may be painted over with a camel's hair brush.

Or if this same kind of burn be very extensive it

may be bathed with warm turpentine, then dredged with flour and wrapped in warm cotton.

A point which should be kept in view in the immediate treatment of all burns, is to protect them *at once* carefully from the air ; all the above methods of treatment have that end in view, except the first, in which cold applications are directed.

If the burn be very extensive or is accompanied by the formation of blisters, the blisters may be punctured just enough to allow the liquid to escape, and flour sprinkled thickly over by means of a common flour dredger ; over this cotton batting of equal thickness must be laid ; a second, a third layer must be laid over this according to the profuseness of the discharge. The whole to be retained in its place by a bandage lightly applied.

If a druggist's shop be near at hand, have a mixture prepared consisting of two parts of collodion and one of castor oil ; puncture the blisters, apply with the camel's hair brush two or three coats of this, then dredge lightly with flour and cover with carded cotton. A case of this kind under the writer's care, the burn being very extensive and severe, and attended with great prostration, by this application ran its course from beginning to end without the *least pain*, or the pain ceasing as soon as the application was made. The collodion and castor oil form an effectual protection from the air, and is very soothing, while the ether which the collodion contains acts as a direct sedative to the pain.

It is to be borne in mind in the treatment of all the above cases that the dressings after having been once applied, are not to be changed for several days except by the direction of the physician, except in cases in which medical assistance cannot be obtained.

Severe burns are frequently attended with fainting or collapse, cold extremities, pale face, &c. ; in such cases give a little brandy or wine.

Choking. Foreign Bodies and Substances in the Throat.

Foreign bodies in the throat either produce irritation or hard coughing, or choking, or find their way down the throat, or are coughed up of themselves.

If the body which gets into the throat be small or sharp, as a fish bone, a pin, make the patient swallow a good mouthful of bread crumb, or it may sometimes be carried down by making the patient swallow a plentiful draught of water or what is better the white of an egg, followed if necessary by a second.

Sometimes if the foreign body be lodged in the *upper* part of the throat it may be visible. In such a case direct some one to hold the tongue with a spoon, and regardless of the attempts to vomit, thrust the finger into the back part of the throat, if it can be reached, and carefully remove the substance, taking care not to lacerate the surrounding parts.

Or a long skein of silk forming a great number of nooses may be pushed down the back part of the throat, the tongue being held with a spoon, keeping hold of one end of the skein. In this manner the sharp body may sometimes be caught and drawn up.

If none of these measures are sufficient an emetic of Sulphate of Zinc must be given; 15 grains will be sufficient for an adult; for the doses for children and infants, see pages IX–X.

If the substance lodged in the throat be a large soft substance as a piece of meat, try to excite vomiting by the means above mentioned. Sometimes a smart blow on the middle of the back just below the neck will dislodge it. If it cannot be thus dislodged (if the patient can hardly breathe do not wait for an emetic of sulphate of zinc to operate,) and medical assistance cannot be speedily obtained, in either of the two classes of substances mentioned, take a large goose quill, push the feathered part into the throat, first having oiled it, directing it well backwards, *so that it may not enter the wind pipe*, which lies in *front* of the throat; then in the first class of substances mentioned, twirl it rapidly about so as to disengage it; in the second, try to push the substance if it be soft, down into the throat aud stomach. Large, hard, angular bodies, as bone, glass, can be removed generally only by extraction; though even in these cases, if medical assistance cannot be obtained, the skein of silk may be employed, followed if this be ineffectual, by an emetic.

Concussion—"Stunning."

Concussion of the brain is a shock given it by some mechanical violence, as a blow, a fall, &c., and is attended with a weakening, or loss of bodily or mental power. Its symptoms vary according to the shock, from giddiness and stupefaction with vomiting, to complete insensibility and stupor. Sometimes the patient can be roused for a moment, becoming immediately insensible again, perhaps after a while partly recovering his senses; in more severe cases it being impossible to arouse the patient, the body becoming pale and cold, the pulse and breathing feeble and all the symptoms of prostration existing.

In severe concussion there are two principal stages. The first is that of collapse or insensibility, the patient may die in this stage without ever becoming conscious. The second is when *reaction* sets in, or the natural powers begin to return, the pulse rising, the breathing becoming stronger and partial or complete consciousness returning.

TREATMENT.—In the first stage, *generally*, do nothing; place. the patient on his back and await the result, particularly do not interfere if he can be roused and is at all sensible, and the collapse be only partial. If however there is great coldness, paleness, complete insensibility which *lasts* a long time, and there are no signs of returning animation, an attempt should be made to being on reaction. Do this by applying warmth to the surface of the body, placing bottles of hot water or bricks under the arms, friction to the chest and abdomen. If these produce no effect give injections containing turpentine, five or six teaspoonfuls beaten up with the yolk of an egg and mixed with water; camphor may be held to the nostrils or a handkerchief sprinkled with ammonia may be passed before the nostrils, not too freely however as it may injure the patient.

As soon as there are signs of returning animation or *reaction* as it is termed technically, or as soon as they have fully set in, do *nothing* except to put the patient on his back, with his head a little elevated; if he be very weak a little gruel or tea may be given. If collapse should threaten to set in again, as it sometimes does, give a little wine and water. Sometimes however the reaction sets in with *too much* violence, the face becoming flushed and the vessels of the head and neck, and the pulse, full and throbbing ; the eyes may be bloodshot, there may be fever, pain in the head, or delirium. In such a case there is danger of inflammation of the brain, and the patient should be placed in a cool darkened room ; cold water should be kept applied to the head, a dose of castor oil should be given, followed by the administration of ***Verat. Vir.*** and ***Bell.*** in alternation, an hour or two apart.

DOSE.—Each of these medicines to be prepared by mixing five drops in half a tumbler of water ; the dose is a teaspoonful.

Finally, do not do too much in this kind of accident. The measures directed above are all that should be attempted except by a physician, and often even, then ; as there is generally an inclination to do too much in these cases, to bleed, to pour stimulants down the patient's throat, &c.

Drowning.

If after the body is taken from the water there are any signs of life, or the breathing have not ceased entirely, employ all possible means to promote circulation and warmth. First place the body with the face downward with the wrist under the forehead.

Cleanse the mouth from froth, mucus, &c.; strip it of its wet clothing, wipe it dry; rub it with dry cloths, hot flannels, or employ friction with the hand; apply bottles of hot water, or heated bricks under the arm pits, to the feet, and to the pit of the stomach; as soon as the signs of returning life are well marked or the patient seems reviving, put the body in a warm bed, or if that be not at hand cover it with as much spare clothing as can be obtained from the by-standers.

An injection containing five or six teaspoonfuls of spirits of turpentine beaten up with the yolk of an egg and mixed with a pint of warm water, or an injection containing a little brandy may also be administered.

When, however, the *warm bath* can be obtained, it is preferable to all other means of restoring circulation and warmth. When the patient can swallow, a little wine and water, or weak brandy or coffee may be given. The patient should be kept in bed and a disposition to sleep encouraged.

But *if there are no signs of breathing and life seem extinct*, resort at once to *artificial respiration*. first having stripped off the wet clothes, and placed the body with the face downwards. Do this, unless the weather be severe, *on the spot*. It is performed in the following manner:

Mode of producing Artificial Respiration:

1. Place the patient on the face upon a table, then turn the body on the side and a little beyond, then briskly on the face or breast again, and so from the side to the face alternately once about every four or five seconds. The side on which the patient is turned should be varied occasionally.

2. Each time the body is placed on the face, make uniform but firm pressure *between and below the shoulder blades, on each side of the spine,* removing the pressure immediately before turning the body on the side.

3. The head should project a little over the edge of the table and the finger or a feather should be occasionally thrust into the back part of the throat to excite vomiting, and from time to time try to excite respiration by passing a handkerchief moistened with hartshorn before the nostrils, or by exciting the nostrils with snuff.

During the whole time rub the limbs upwards with handkerchiefs, flannels, &c., and keep the body as warm as possible. Injections containing brandy or turpentine may be also given, prepared as directed above; or injections of very warm water may be given.

If after long continued efforts there are no signs of returning animation, substitute in place of the artificial respiration, vigorous friction all over with dry flannel, three or four men relieving each other every half hour. From time to time the artificial respiration may be resorted to again.

In the case in which animation has been restored after the longest period of submersion, a period of *fourteen minutes*, respiration was brought about by this last method, (the friction.) Not the slightest appearance of animation however manifested itself, until these efforts had been continued with the utmost industry for *eight hours and a half*, when feeble respiration commenced ; the friction was made in this case by relays of four men who relieved each other every half hour.

This case shows that the efforts at restoration should not be too soon abandoned, but should be persevered in for hours, even though life should seem quite gone. Few cases however in which the body has been submerged for so long a time, can be attended with such happy results as this. It is very doubtful whether restoration can be hoped for if the body have been immersed more than fourteen minutes, though a number of cases, not however, well authenticated, have been reported of restoration after immersion for a much longer period.

Part of the above directions for the treatment of cases of drowning, have been taken from the directions of the Royal Humane Society. The following directions from the same source should also be care fully observed:

1. Send for medical assistance and dry clothing.
2. Avoid rough usage.
3. Avoid using the warm bath *for too long a time*.
4. Do not let persons crowd about the body.

Substances and Bodies in the Ears.

Children frequently get foreign bodies of different kinds, as peas, cherry stones, bits of pencil, &c., into the ear; or a fly may find its way into the ear and occasion great distress.

TREATMENT.—If the substance be full in view and it can be easily grasped by a small pair of forceps, it may be extricated by them. Or it may sometimes be easily removed if within reach, by a knitting needle or wire, the point being slightly bent. No attempts should however be made to extract it by these means, unless it can be done without much force. When it cannot be thus easily removed, the simplest and most effective method consists in the forcible injection of warm water into the ear, by means of a good sized syringe. This if continued a sufficient length of time, will rarely fail to bring away the offending substance.

Freezing, and the Effects of Severe Cold.

If any of the extremities or any part of the body be frozen, rub it briskly with snow or iced water, and, as sensibility returns, cold water of the usual temperature may be substituted and the friction made somewhat more briskly. Do not go near the fire, but let the applications be made in a cold room or on the spot where the freezing occurs; the sooner the better. Keep the frozen part cool and avoid a high temperature until the sensibility of the frozen part is restored and it seems to have recovered its natural condition; the parts most liable to be frozen are those most remote from the heart, the great organ of circulation, as the hands, feet, ears, nose, and heels; the circulation in these parts being feebler and they being also the most exposed.

The first visible effect of severe cold is to change the affected part to a dull red color, as the cold increases in severity or if it continue, the part gradually loses color and becomes white, pale, and insensible. This is the appearance presented by a part which is "frost bitten."

2. *Complete Insensibility from Cold.*—The same principles are to be observed, when a person has become nearly or quite insensible from the effects of severe or long continued cold. If there be complete insensibility, plunge the body, if it can be done

speedily, into a bath of *ice water*, and suffer it to remain for two or three minutes, after which take it out, rub it with snow and proceed as hereafter directed. If such a bath cannot be speedily obtained, or *if there be not complete insensibility*, place the body in a cool bed in a cool room, and rub it with snow from head to feet; an injection containing 5 or 6 teaspoonfuls of spirits of turpentine beaten up with the yolk of an egg and mixed with water, or an injection containing a little brandy may be given; if there be complete insensibility, breathe from time to time into the patient's mouth. As soon as there are any signs of returning sensibility and warmth, substitute for the snow, cold water of the ordinary temperature, and continue the friction. As soon as the patient can swallow, a little warm wine and water very weak may be given, and when sensibility and warmth are somewhat restored, frictions with dry flannels and furs may be employed.

After a while, when a natural condition seems to have been brought about, the patient may be laid in a room slightly warmed, wrapped in flannel or fur, a little warm gruel may be given, and gentle friction made from time to time with the hand.

Finally, in the treatment of the effects of cold these two rules should be kept in view: 1. *The applications should at first be as cold as possible*

2. *The temperature of the applications should be gradually increased as the part recovers its natural condition.*

Hanging.

Where suicide has been attempted by hanging, loosen all the clothing about the neck and chest, then if the breathing have not ceased, simply place the patient on the back with the head raised ; though if there seem to be much fullness of the head, give a dose or two of Aconite and Belladonna in alternation, if they can be swallowed.

If however the breathing have ceased and life seem extinct, having loosened the clothing about the neck and chest, resort at once to artificial respiration as directed on page 104, and dash cold water frequently on the face and chest. Hartshorn, snuff, &c., may be also applied occasionally to the nostrils, and the throat tickled with a feather.

Artificial respiration may also be made occasionally by placing a pipe in the nostril and blowing through it ; or a tube may be made, by rolling up a piece of paper, or the muzzle of a bellows may be introduced into one nostril, closing the other with the finger.

Breathe or blow gently once in four or five seconds, each time you blow or breathe, pressing the prominence known as "Adam's apple," firmly back. The blowing through the nose should not however be resorted to unless the artificial respiration first described should prove ineffectual.

If respiration after having been once brought on should cease again, the same measures must be repeated.

After the patient has recovered somewhat. put him to bed and wrap him up warmly.

Injury from Lightning.

When a person has been stunned or struck by lightning, unless there are *unmistakeable* signs of death, strip off the clothing and dash cold water freely upon the body, for ten or fifteen minutes. Diligent friction should also be employed, injections containing turpentine or brandy should be administered, and ammonia applied freely to the nostrils. Should the cold water not bring on some signs of respiration, artificial respiration should be resorted to as described on page 104, and the stimulants continued from time to time.

Sprains, Strains.

A sprain may be an injury of a very serious nature, sometimes requiring a much longer time for its cure than a broken limb. It is commonly attended with redness, pain, and impaired motion of the affected part; in severe cases there are also swelling and heat.

The injury consists in the forcible stretching or laceration of some of the fibres either of the muscles or ligaments.

TREATMENT.—If there be much heat in the injured part, keep it wet until the heat has somewhat subsided, with a mixture composed of one part of alcohol to two parts of water.

If there is not a great deal of heat, keep the part covered with a linen cloth wet with a mixture of Arnica and water in the proportion of three teaspoonfuls of the former to a tumbler of the latter. Internally *Arnica and Rhus* should be taken according to the directions for doses, contained in the introduction.

The part should be kept at rest. If the wrist be injured, the arm should be supported by a sling, if the foot, the leg should be kept raised up on a chair.

Suffocation from Smoke, the Fumes of Charcoal, Poisonous Gases, &c.

A person suffocated by the smoke or the fumes of charcoal, should be removed at once to the air, cold water should be dashed freely over the head and chest, and hartshorn, snuff, &c., applied to the nostrils. If the remedies are not soon succeeded by some signs of returning animation, artificial respiration as described on page 104 must be employed.

Bottles of hot water or heated bricks may also be applied to the feet and under the arm pits. When there are signs of recovery, place the body in a warm bed, in a room in which there is a good free passage of air. Cold acid drinks may also be given, as lemonade, claret, &c.

Sun Stroke—Coup de Soleil.

The symptoms attending this accident are owing to nervous exhaustion. The clothing about the neck and chest should be loosened ; cold water should be dashed freely upon the head, neck and chest, hartshorn occasionally applied to the nostrils, until consciousness returns ; then administer brandy or wine liberally, and keep cold water or ice applied to the head, and as soon as the patient recovers a little nourishment should be given.

Wounds, Cuts.

A cut may or may not be accompanied by profuse bleeding. If it be, the measures for stopping it described on pages 89–95 must be resorted to.

Incised wounds, or, as they are more commonly called, cuts, are, however, generally accompanied by considerable bleeding. If they are not, or if the bleeding be pretty effectually checked, or the wound be slight, it may be treated as hereafter directed. *Un-*

less, however, the cut is small, or even if it be on a part of the body where a scar would be unsightly, unless medical assistance cannot be obtained, it should be dressed by a surgeon.

1. Stop the bleeding as directed on pages 89–95.

2. Remove all foreign substances as dirt, sand, bits of glass, &c., from the wound. This may be done by the fingers or by washing the wound thoroughly with cold water.

3. Then, if the edges of the wound are not close together, bring them together, so that they will fit *smoothly*, and confine them so by strips of arnica plaster, or any kind of adhesive plaster, placed across the wound, leaving a small space between the strips.

Lacerated and Contused Wounds.

These wounds are caused by some blunt instrument or by some object which tears the surface. In lacerated wounds, the edges are jagged and irregular, in contused they are bruised.

Neither of these wounds is accompanied by much bleeding; if there be any, however, it must be checked as directed on pages 89–95, and the wound must be washed as clean as possible, and all foreign substances removed by means of warm water and a sponge.

Lacerated wounds cannot generally be made to heal readily and smoothly by bringing their edges together, as in incised wounds. The edges however must be brought together as smoothly as possible, and if it be small, plaster may be applied as directed when treating of incised wounds.

If however, it be large or very irregular, keep linen cloths applied, wet with cold water. If it be a contused or *bruised* wound, and the surrounding parts are swollen and tense, arnica may be added to the water, in the proportion of 30 drops to a tumbler full. After the bleeding has ceased, if there be much prostration, warm water may be substituted for cold.

Wounds and Injuries from Fire Arms.

A gun or pistol may be loaded only with powder and wadding, and yet produce a severe lacerated wound. A wound of this character should be treated according to the directions given above.

If the ball enter deeply and either goes through the part or lodges in it, and is followed by bleeding, measures should first be taken to stop it. (See directions on page 89.) If the wound be not deep firm pressure with the fingers on its upper and lower edge should be employed. If this fail, resort to the tourniquet, or if the ball lodge deep in one of the limbs and is *not* followed by bleeding, the tourniquet should invariably be applied, as severe hæmorrhage may be going on internally. Profuse hæmorrhage from gunshot wounds is, however, not common, unless some large vessel has been wounded.

Punctured Wounds

Are such as are made by any sharp *pointed* instrument; they are generally deep. The treatment in regard to bleeding, and the after treatment should be the same directed for wounds from fire arms.

SYNOPSIS.

General Affections in which the Remedies Contained in the Case are useful.

Aconite.—In fever and in all complaints accompanied by fever. It may be given alone, or in alternation with any other remedy.

Aloes.—In dysentery or diarrhœa, accompanied by bilious stools and burning at the anus.

Arnica.—For bruises, sprains, dislocations. It may be used both internally and as an external application.

Arsenicum.—Is useful in colds accompanied by pains about the eyes and forehead ; in disorders of the stomach, and dyspepsia accompanied by nausea, vomiting, thirst,or burning ; in watery diarrhœa ; in headaches from cold or indigestion ; *sick* headaches ; may be given in alternation with Nux, Bell, or Coloc, &c.

Belladonna.—In scarlet fever, in sore throats with difficulty of swallowing, particularly if there be much *redness* of the throat ; in headaches accompanied by throbbing, pains in the eyes and temples, *fullness* of the head, threatened apoplexy ; convulsions of infants ; pains in the ear.

BRYONIA.—In headaches accompanied with soreness of the head; bad taste in the mouth; derangement of the liver; fevers accompanied by prostration, exhaustion, and general soreness.

CHAMOMILLA.—In colicky pains of infants with green, watery or slimy stools; in threatened miscarriage and in false labor pains.

COLCHICUM. In rheumatic pains particularly if they affect the joints; aching in the limbs and bones from cold; sharp, rheumatic pains in the chest.

COLOCYNTH.—Watery diarrhœa with or without crampy pains in the bowels; crampy pains or cramps in the legs or arms; colicky pains without diarrhœa. In threatened miscarriage and in false labor pains.

DULCAMARA.—In watery or slimy diarrhœa proceeding from cold; with or without slight colicky pains.

GELSEMINUM.—In fever accompanied by great prostration and debility, with nervous exhaustion, with or without chilliness or perspiration; neuralgic pains in various parts of the head and back of the head and shoulders, occurring either as the result of cold, being rheumatic or neuralgic in their character, or accompanying febrile conditions. The most ***prominent*** characteristic of the fever and various conditions which call for the use of this remedy, is ***great weakness of the nervous, or muscular system.***

HEPAR SULPHUR.—Colds in the head; accumulation of phlegm in the throat; constant inclination to clear the throat; hacking cough. May be given in alternation with *Stib.*, *Nux*, or *Kali.*

HAMAMELIS.—In dysentery with bloody stools, and straining at the anus.

HYOSCYAMUS.—In convulsions of infants; in dry, hard fits of coughing, sleeplessness, nervousness. May be used in alternation with *Bell.*, *Stibium*, *Nux*, &c.

IGNATIA.—Nervous headaches; hysterical affections; headache with great irritability; headaches accompanied with soreness; convulsions of infants; pains in the temples. May be given in alternation with *Ars.*, *Bell.*, &c.

IPECAC.—In dysentery accompanied by much *straining* at the anus; in simple diarrhœa attended with nausea.

JALAP.—In diarrhœa of infants proceeding from cold, and accompanied by colicky pains.

KALI BICHROMATE.—Useful in colds in the head; cough, with hoarseness and loss of voice; loose cough; cough from accumulation of mucus in the throat.

KALI HYDRIODIDE.—Coughs from cold, worse night and morning; loose cough, with rattling of mucus in the chest; running from the eyes and nose; dry coughs. May be given in alternation with *Hyos.*, *Nux*, *Stibium*, &c.

MERCURIUS CORROSIVUS.—In dysentery with bloody passages; discharges of pure blood or bloody mucus; straining and burning at the anus; cutting pains in the bowels with the dysentery.

MERCURIUS DULCIS.—Hard, colicky pains in the bowels, attended with cold perspiration or with *soreness* of the bowels; in dry coughs, with soreness of the chest. May be alternated with *Nux* or *Coloc.*

MERCURIUS PROTIODIDE.—Ulcerated sore throat with difficulty of swallowing; swelling and enlargement of the glands of the throat. May be given in alternation with *Stibium*

MERCURIUS SOLUBILIS.—In sore throat accompanied with difficulty of swallowing; swelling of the glands of the throat; diphtheria; in pains of the limbs and bones from taking cold, *if accompanied by perspiration;* headaches from derangement of the liver; diarrhœa, with green, slimy, or jelly-like passages, bloody stools, soreness, straining or burning at the anus; white, clay-colored stools; brown, watery passages; pains in the face, teeth, or ears from cold; summer complaints of children. It may be given in alternation, as required, with *Stibium* or *Bell.*, for sore throat; with

Bell, for pains in the face or teeth; with *Veratrum*, *Colocynth*, or *Ipecac*, for diarrhœa, dysentery; with *Aconite* or *Stibium* for pains affecting the system after taking cold.

NUX VOMICA.—Headaches from derangement of liver or stomach; sick headaches; colicky pains; indigestion, nausea; nervous headaches; dry, hacking cough; cough worse morning and evening; convulsions. May be given alternately with whatever other remedy is indicated.

OPIUM.—In apoplexy with stupor, drowsiness, &c.; in convulsions of children.

PHOSPHORUS.—In colds accompanied by soreness in the chest; cough accompanied by soreness and burning in the windpipe. *Merc. Sol.* or *Merc. Dulc.* will generally be found *more* useful in these troubles.

PODOPHYLLUM.—This acts upon the liver to such an extent, that it is often called the "vegetable mercury." It is suited particularly to bilious conditions; to headaches proceeding from inaction or congestion of the liver; to such bilious derangements as are characterized by constipation, yellow skin, yellow or white tongue, nausea, yellowish tinge of the eyes. In slight bilious attacks from cold, accompanied by chilliness or shivering with or without fever, it will be found, given in alternation with Aconite, of great service.

PULSATILLA.—In delay or suppression of the monthly sickness. May be given in this affection in alternation with ***Nux, Aconite,*** or any other remedy that may be indicated. Useful in dyspepsia with nausea, bad taste in the mouth, headache from eating rich food, sick headache. More suitable for women and persons with light hair and blue eyes.

RHEUM.—In diarrhœa of infants accompanied by colicky pains, with fits of screaming, &c.; green fermented-looking or sour-smelling passages. Give in alternation, if necessary, with ***Coloc., Verat.*** or ***Cham.***

RHUS.—Rheumatic pains and lameness; aching in the limbs; sharp pains in the limbs or *chest.* May be given in alternation with ***Colch.*** or ***Acon.***

SAMBUCUS.—In false croup ("Miller's Asthma")

SPONGIA.—In hoarseness with or without burning in the larynx. Give in alternation with ***Stib., Merc. Sol.,*** or any other remedy that may be required.

STIBIUM.—In all catarrhal affections; chilliness, aching in the bones, &c., after taking cold; sore throat, with or without difficulty of swallowing; cough; cold in the head; measles. May be given in alternation with ***Merc. Sol.*** or ***Merc. Protiod.,*** in sore throats; ***Merc., Dulc., Kali, Nux,*** &c., in coughs; *Ac.*, *Merc. Sol.*, in rheumatic pains after taking cold.

SULPHATE OF ZINC.—To be used as an emetic.

SULPHUR.—In constipation, piles.

TARTAR EMETIC —In croup.

VERATRUM.—In diarrhœa with or without colicky pains; thin watery passages; dark or light-colored passages.

VERATRUM VIRIDE.—This remedy is a more important one, and suited to a greater *variety* of fevers, than Aconite. In scarlatina, in bronchial affections, in affections of the chest accompanied by fever, in pleurisy, pneumonia, &c., it is invaluable. In fever produced by teething, it is useful; and in simple fever, is as reliable as any other. In disorders of the brain characterised by *great fullness*, it is more serviceable than even Belladonna. It is particularly applicable when the fever is *high*, the pulse hard and full, and where there is *great excitement of the circulation* generally; it controls this state better than any other known remedy. The more violent the fever, the more suitable is Veratrum Viride.

Any one of the above remedies may be given in alternation with any other one which seems suited to the nature of the case.

APPENDIX.

Fevers.

A Fever may be considered to exist when the pulse is quickened, when there is a sensation of chilliness, furred tongue, and hot skin. These symptoms are the ones most commonly present, though there are others which very frequently accompany it, among which may be mentioned headache; pain in the back; an aching, sore, and bruised feeling throughout the system; debility; constipation and high-colored urine. Often, instead of a simple chilliness, will occur a *violent* chill, as severe as that of intermittent fever. These various symptoms may be produced by a simple cold, and may be easily controlled, running their course probably in a few days, and constituting *simple* or *transient* fever. In children, these simple fevers may be produced by teething, or may result from indigestion.

The remedies indicated in the treatment are as follows. In case the pulse is high and the skin burning, *Aconite* should be made an important remedy; and in case there is chilliness, soreness, aching in the limbs, and coated tongue, *Merc. Sol.* should be given in alternation with it.

Should the febrile symptoms not be relieved by Aconite, *Veratrum Viride* will probably control them.

Gelseminum and *Bryonia* are applicable where there is excessive lassitude, headache, and general soreness.

In the simple fever of children, *Aconite* will generally be found the most useful remedy. *Mercurius Sol.* may be given in alternation with it, if the fever seem to proceed from a cold. In case Aconite do not allay the fever, *Veratrum Viride* may be used in place of it.

In fever from teething, *Aconite* should be administered, *Belladonna* being given in alternation with it, if there be much heat of the head; and *Cham.* and *Aconite,* if there be much fretfulness and peevishness.

In fever from indigestion, give *Aconite* and *Pulsatilla;* and if there be constipation, produce a movement of the bowels by means of an injection.

In some cases, the heat, headache, and chill may indicate the approach of some more serious disease than simple fever, as typhus, typhoid, pneumonia, &., in which case the remedies above indicated will be of but little use—the early approaches of these diseases being intricate, and sometimes even milder than those of simple fevers

Hysteria—"Hysterics."

This disease, though not often attended with danger, is commonly very distressing. The symptoms which characterize an attack are almost innumerable, and often simulate the most serious diseases; indeed, there is scarcely a disease which they may not resemble. The most common symptoms are a sensation of choking; a feeling as if there were a ball or plug in the throat; a feeling as if there were a ball rolling about in the bowels, and rising up to the chest and throat; rumbling and eructations of wind; a sense of tightness and constriction of the chest. The patient feels hardly able to breathe, and as if she would suffocate. There may be weeping alternated with laughter; great restlessness; palpitation of the heart; often screaming. The patient is inconsolable, and will not listen to any reason; the face is purple, and the patient looks as if she were strangling; struggles violently, so that it may require several persons to hold her; throws herself about; there are pains in the chest; sometimes there is almost complete insensibility, with slow and heavy breathing. The attack may last for hours.

DIAGNOSIS.—This will be rendered more easy by ascertaining if the patient has been subject to attacks of Hysteria. The disease for which a severe attack of Hysteria is most likely to be mistaken is epilepsy. In the latter disease, there is frothing at the mouth; the eyes have a fixed, dull, protruded look; the jaws are tightly closed; the face is much distorted. In Hysteria, if the eye-lid be raised, the eye will be seen to be bright and natural, though it may be fixed; the face is not often distorted, nor is the breathing so very difficult as in epilepsy, as the patient succeeds now and then in taking a long, full breath; there is seldom loss of consciousness, the patient, when the attack is over, remembering everything that has passed, though she may *seem* unconscious during the attack.

In epilepsy, the struggles of the patient are generally less violent.

TREATMENT.—During the attack give plenty of fresh air; apply burnt feathers to the nose; loosen the dress; and if the attack be *very severe*, cold water may be poured in a stream from a height upon the head and *face*, in spite of the screams of the patient, care being taken, however, to cover her, so that the wetting will be confined to the head and face. This may seem severe treatment, but there are cases in which the patient is so excited, and the attack is so bad, that nothing else which can be given by non-medical persons will do so much good, or will break up the attack. It should be poured upon the head and face until the paroxysm gives way. Assafœtida, Valerian, &c., are overrated.

CAUSES, ETC.—Hysterical attacks always depend upon some derangement of the health; indigestion; want of exercise; anything which exhausts the system, or impairs the health; but most frequently upon some disorder of the uterus, or derangement or disorder of the monthly sickness. Females from fifteen to forty years of age are most liable to the disease. The treatment during the intervals of the attack should be directed to the cure of whatever derangement of the system the attacks may depend upon.

Scarlatina or Scarlet Fever—"Scarlet Rash."

I refer to this disease here, not that people may treat it—as the mildest cases should be placed under a physician's care—but because there are many erroneous ideas prevalent concerning it. One of these is, that Scarlatina is a very mild and harmless form of Scarlet Fever, and that Scarlet Rash is still different from either. The truth is, that they are all one and the same disease. Scarlatina is simply the *Latin* name for Scarlet Fever or Scarlet

Rash—the common or vulgar appellation of the disease. It is not unusual for mothers to say, "Oh, it is only scarlatina," regarding it as an affair of but little moment; while the mildest case is not only capable of producing the most virulent form of the disease, but is very liable to be followed by dropsy or by some affection of the throat or hearing.

Scarlatina is often ushered in by vomiting; this is accompanied or soon followed by chilliness, shivering, back-ache, fever, which are usually followed on the second or third day by an eruption of fine red points, which become so numerous as to unite, forming one general red surface; the pulse is generally very rapid, and the temperature of the surface high. The eruption first makes its appearance upon the face, neck, and arms; then upon the trunk; and finally upon the legs.

In the mildest form, the fever and redness of the skin are almost the only abnormal conditions present, the throat being but slightly, or not at all, affected. In the more severe forms, the disease may exist in various degrees of intensity, sometimes producing ulcerated sore throat and inflammation of various parts of the ear, and sometimes affecting almost every tissue of the body, disorganizing the blood, producing swelling of the joints, congestion of the kidneys and brain, and in the form known as *malignant* scarlatina, overwhelming the system with the intensity of its poison, and rapidly extinguishing the vital powers.

The *fever* in all cases lasts at least five or six days. The mild form, with care, almost always progresses favorably, but still demands watchfulness. After the *mildest* attack, the patient should be kept warm, and not be allowed to go into the open air sooner than three or four weeks.

TREATMENT.—*Verat. Vir.* and *Bell.* should be given and in case the throat be affected, *Bell.* and *Merc. Sol.*

It is superfluous to recommend more remedies; as in cases at all severe, the selection of the proper medicines demands experience and careful discrimination.

Measles.

Is a disease accompanied by fever, an eruption upon the skin, and affecting principally the mucous membrane of the eyes, nose, air passages, and the bowels. It is preceded by running at the eyes and nose, hoarseness, and by symptoms of cold generally, and is often accompanied by nausea and vomiting.

These symptoms are usually accompanied by fever; and in about four days an eruption makes its appearance upon the face, neck, and upper extremities, consisting at first only of a few small spots, resembling flea-bites. These increase in number and in size, and finally become larger and of a dark red color. Generally, the patches are not so numerous as to conceal the healthy skin, as is the case in scarlet fever. The eruption commonly appears on the fifth day upon the trunk, and on the sixth day upon the lower extremities. The fever and eruption do not abate for six or seven days. Diarrhœa is a common accompaniment of the advanced stage of the disease. Though Measles is generally a very tractable disease, it is sometimes very serious. The eruption may be slow in making its appearance, the poison irritating the system in various ways, and producing severe bronchitis, congestion of the lungs, stupor, or convulsions. Sometimes it is accompanied by great prostration, or the eruption may be abundant and of an unhealthy color. Vomiting and diarrhœa may be excessive. In young infants, it is often serious.

The treatment of Measles consists in the treatment of the various symptoms as they occur. In the first stage, for the catarrhal condition, with fever, shivering, ***Veratrum Vir.*** an ***Mercurius Sol.*** may be given, an hour apart. After a few doses of the latter have been given, ***Kali Bich.*** may be substituted for it. In case the catarrh affects the chest or throat, the remedies mentioned on page 21 should be given. The fever of Measles cannot be shortened, but must run its course. Sometimes the non-appearance of the rash wlll produce convulsion, and must be treated as directed on page 34.

INDEX.

With the Abbreviations of the Medicines suited to each Complaint and Condition

---

For Doses, Manner of Administration, &c., consult pages ix, x, xii. For Description of the Effects and Uses of the various Remedies mentioned in this work, see Synopsis, p. 116.

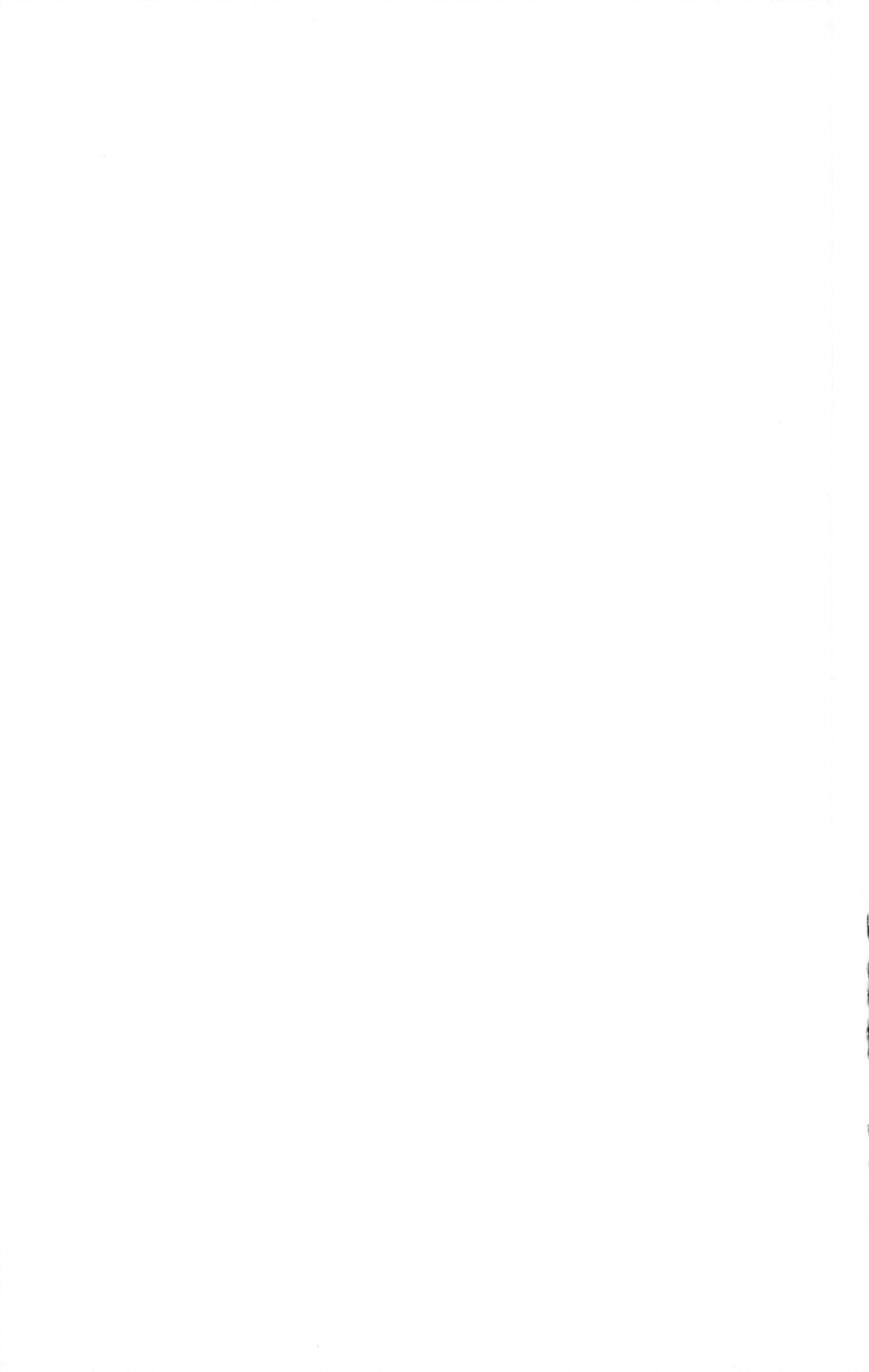

www.ingramcontent.com/pod-product-compliance
Lightning Source LLC
LaVergne TN
LVHW021415110826
845150LV00007B/1934